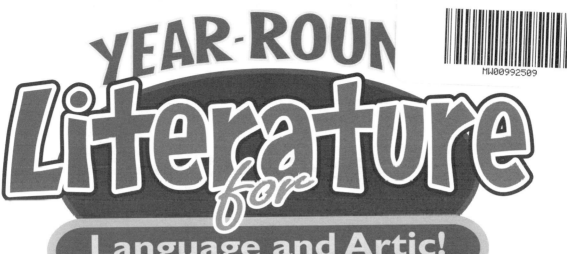

# YEAR-ROUND Literature for Language and Artic!

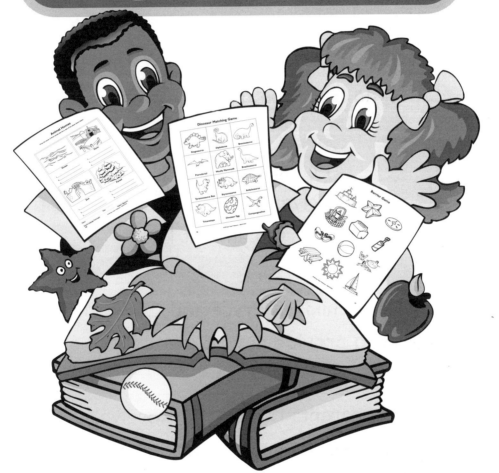

## Written by Rochelle Wilson
## Illustrated by Tony Mitchell

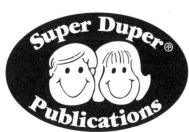

Super Duper® Publications

www.superduperinc.com
Post Office Box 24997, Greenville, South Carolina 29616 USA
1-800-277-8737 • Fax 1-800-978-7379
Email: custserv@superduperinc.com

#BK-272
ISBN 1-58650-074-0

# Dedication

This book is dedicated to:


My Lord Jesus Christ,
Who has given me all that I have.


My husband Dave,
Who gives me his love and
Support in all that I do.


My children Bryce and Carly,
Who provide new joys each day.


My parents Darrel and Roselyn,
Who helped me become who I am today.


Thank you all!

#BK-272  Year-Round Literature  •  ©1999 Super Duper® Publications  •  1-800-277-8737  •  www.superduperinc.com

# Introduction

*Year-Round Literature for Language and Artic!* takes an innovative approach to articulation and language therapy, combining popular children's books with the use of common and interesting themes. These themes, having been tested in the classroom with hundreds of students, have been designed to help speech-language pathologists remediate articulation problems and improve language skills in their students. Each of the themes in this book include theme-specific:

- Articulation Words
- Pictures/Activities
- Story Patterns
- Reading/Activities
- Language Questions
- Games
- Worksheets

The thematic approach to therapy not only provides continuity in learning, but also makes therapy exciting for both students and the therapist. When addressing articulation problems, the thematic approach helps students learn their target sound(s) within a context, providing an enriching atmosphere for students to learn correct sound production. When addressing language goals, students are able to learn individual skills, apply them, and then use these skills in a real-life context. The themes create a continuity in therapy sessions that flows throughout each theme's lesson plans.

The following ideas and reproducible pages can help you prepare goal-specific and age-appropriate lesson plans for each of your students. In addition, therapists have found thematic classroom decorations complete the total atmosphere for learning.

Most of all, have fun as you're using *Year-Round Literature for Language and Artic!*

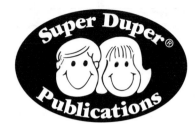

Date _____

Dear Parents/Helpers,

We are now studying a unit about the _____ in order to address your child's speech and language goals. There will be several activities that your child will participate in dealing with <u>the</u>_____. These activities will be tailored to help your child improve his or her speech and language.

In addition, some practice pages will be sent home so that your child will carry over the skills learned in speech class into other life settings.

Thank you for your support and help at home.

Sincerely,

_____

Speech-Language Pathologist

#BK-272  Year-Round Literature  •  ©1999 Super Duper® Publications  •  1-800-277-8737  •  www.superduperinc.com

# Table of Contents

Fall . . . . . . . . . . . . . . . . . . . . . . . . . . . . 1–20

Winter . . . . . . . . . . . . . . . . . . . . . 21–40

Spring . . . . . . . . . . . . . . . . . . . . . 41–60

Summer . . . . . . . . . . . . . . . . . . . . 61–82

Dinosaur. . . . . . . . . . . . . . . . . . . 83–102

Circus. . . . . . . . . . . . . . . . . . . . 103–124

Our Bodies. . . . . . . . . . . . . . . . 125–146

Farm . . . . . . . . . . . . . . . . . . . . . 147–168

Our Town . . . . . . . . . . . . . . . . 169–188

Ocean. . . . . . . . . . . . . . . . . . . . 189–207

# Book List

## Fall

Red Leaf, Yellow Leaf, by Lois Ehlert..................................................................... p. 8
The Apple Pie Tree, by Zoe Hall ...................................................................... p. 9
Sun, Snow, Stars and Sky, by Catherine and Laurence Anholt ...................... p. 10

## Winter

The Mitten, by Jan Brett .................................................................................. p. 28
Snowballs, by Lois Ehlert ............................................................................... p. 29
The Snowy Day, by Ezra Keats ...................................................................... p. 30

## Spring

The Spring Snowman, by Jill Barnes ............................................................... p. 48
Hopper Hunts for Spring, by Marcus Pfister .................................................. p. 49
The Very Hungry Caterpillar, by Eric Carle.................................................... p. 50

## Summer

Sunflower House, by Eve Bunting .................................................................. p. 68
How I Spent My Summer Vacation, by Marc Teague ..................................... p. 69
The Relatives Came, by Cynthia Rylant ......................................................... p. 70

## Dinosaurs

Whatever Happened to the Dinosaurs?, by Bernard Most .............................. p. 90
I Met a Dinosaur, by Jan Wahl ....................................................................... p. 91
Can I Have a Stegosaurus Mom? Can I? Please!?, by Louis G. Grambling ..... p. 92

# Book List

## Circus

*Olivia Saves the Circus*, by Ian Falconer ..................................................p. 110
*The Circus Surprise*, by Ralph Fletcher.......................................................p. 111
*The 12 Circus Rings*, by Seymore Chwast ................................................p. 112

## Our Bodies

*From Head to Toe*, by Eric Carle ..............................................................p. 133
*My Hands*, by Aliki...................................................................................p. 134
*Here Are My Hands*, by Bill Martin, Jr. and John Archambault....................p. 135

## Farm

*The Day Jimmy's Boa Ate the Wash*, by Trinka Noble...................................p. 154
*The Big Red Barn*, by Margaret Brown.......................................................p. 155
*Barn Dance*, by Bill Martin, Jr. and John Archambault ...............................p. 156

## Our Town

*Me on the Map*, by Joan Sweeny...............................................................p. 177
*The Adventures of Taxi Dog*, by Debra and Sal Barracca .............................p. 178
*Secret Place*, by Eve Bunting ...................................................................p. 179

## Ocean

*Big Al*, by Andrew Clements ......................................................................p. 196
*The Rainbow Fish*, by Marcus Pfister .........................................................p. 197
*Swimmy*, by Leo Lionni.............................................................................p. 198

# Language and Artic Activities
# for all Theme Units

**Articulation and Vocabulary Word Lists** – Each unit begins with a list of articulation/vocabulary word lists. Words are divided by sound in the initial, medial, and final positions, plus blends. These words are a good resource for articulation and/or vocabulary building activities that relate to the theme of the unit.

**Vocabulary Pictures** – Each unit has vocabulary pictures. These pictures can be cut out and used as vocabulary cards. They may also be used to elicit descriptions of each picture. In addition, students can be asked to sort the pictures into categories such as animals, clothing, food, etc.

## Game Ideas

*   Make two copies of each of the selected pictures and make a matching game.
*   Make copies of and laminate selected cards and put them in a hat. Allow each student to pull a card out and make a sentence about the picture using correct target language and articulation structures.
*   Hide cards around the room and allow each student a turn to find a card and tell about the picture using correct language and articulation structures.

**Story Pattern** – Each unit has a story pattern that should be used with stories in that unit.

## Story Pattern Ideas

*   Have the students look at the front cover of the book and make predictions about what they believe will happen in the story. Then, have the students write or dictate their predictions on the story pattern. As the students are writing, monitor their use of grammatical structures. After writing the prediction, have each student underline any word with his/her sound and read the prediction out loud using his/her good sound. If the students are working on language structures, ask "wh" questions about the prediction and then probe for vocabulary, categories, functions, attributes, and definitions using both the prediction and the illustration from the front cover.
*   After reading the book, have each student sequence the events of the book. Students may verbally dictate or write the sequence of events on the following story pattern. Ask each student to use sequence words, such as first, second, third, and last.
*   After reading the book, go through each page individually with the group. Target specific words and ask the group to think of words that rhyme with the given word from the book. Write the words on the story patterns. Make a goal for the group to have a certain number of rhyming words on the story pattern by the end of class.

 #BK-272  Year-Round Literature  •  ©1999 Super Duper® Publications  •  1-800-277-8737  •  www.superduperinc.com

# Fall

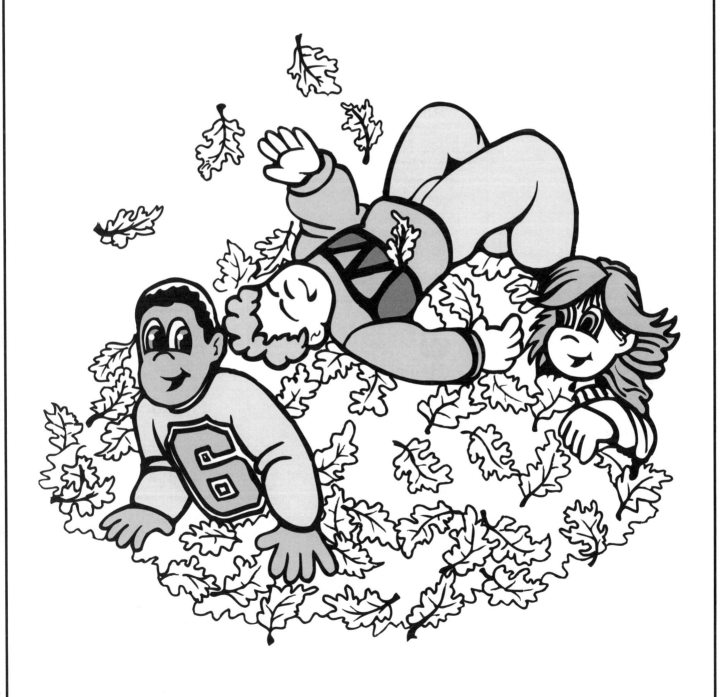

# Fall Articulation & Vocabulary Word Lists

These word lists are a good resource for articulation and/or vocabulary building activities.

## /r/ and /r/ blends

### Initial
rake

red

### Medial
squirrels

turkey

orange

harvest

### Final
sweater

apple cider

campfire

cool weather

September

October

November

December

### Blends
jack-o-lantern

fir tree

nutcracker

scarecrow

crow

trick-or-treat

brown

chrysanthemums

tree

acorn

migrate

maple tree

oak tree

long-sleeved shirt

sycamore tree

spruce tree

birch tree

pine tree

## /s/ and /s/ blends

### Initial
season

September

sycamore tree

### Medial
apple cider

chrysanthemums

December

### Final
nuts

chestnuts

long pants

geese

ghosts

### Blends
sweatshirt

squirrels

scarecrow

school

spruce tree

chestnuts

feast

harvest

sweater

Thanksgiving

long-sleeved shirt

## /z/

### Medial
leaves change colors

### Final
acorns

apples

leaves

birds

Pilgrims

Indians

## /l/ and /l/ blends

### Initial
leaves

long pants

### Medial
jack-o-lantern

apple cider

yellow

chilly

helmet

maple tree

Halloween

Pilgrim

willow tree

### Final
fall

school

football

### Blends
long-sleeved shirt

black cat

cold weather

birds fly south

apples

black cat

elm tree

squirrels

## /k/ and /k/ blends

### Initial
cool weather

campfire

### Medial
acorn

jack-o-lantern

black cat

pumpkin

trick-or-treat

turkey

oak tree

leaves change colors

sycamore tree

jacket

### Final
rake

### Blends
chrysanthemums

squirrels

scarecrow

#BK-272  Year-Round Literature • ©1999 Super Duper® Publications • 1-800-277-8737 • www.superduperinc.com

# Fall Articulation & Vocabulary Word Lists (Cont.)

## /k/ and /k/ blends cont.
### Blends cont.
school
nutcracker
squirrel
Thanksgiving
October

## /g/ and /g/ blends
### Initial
geese
ghost

### Medial
Thanksgiving
dogwood tree

### Blends
migrate
pilgrim

## /th/
### Initial
Thanksgiving
thankful
thermometer

### Medial
cool weather
chrysanthemums

### Final
birds fly south

## /sh/
### Initial
shade tree

### Medial
migration
long-sleeved shirt
ash tree
bushel
sweatshirt

## /ch/
### Initial
chestnuts
chilly

### Medial
leaves change colors
birch tree
wind chill
cool temperature
apple orchard

## /m/ and /m/ blends
### Initial
migrate
maple tree

### Medial
chrysanthemum
sycamore tree

### Final
autumn
Pilgrim

### Blends
September
November
December
pumpkin
campfire
football helmet

## /p/ and /p/ blends
### Initial
pumpkin
pine tree
Pilgrims
poplar tree

### Medial
long pants

### Blends
spruce tree
maple tree
pumpkin

September
apple
apple cider

## /b/ and /b/ blends
### Initial
birds
birch tree
back to school

### Medial
football
October
November
December
football field

### Blends
brown leaves
black cat

## /f/ and /f/ blends
### Initial
feast
football
fir tree

### Medial
football field

### Final
leaf

### Blends
birds fly south

## /v/ and /v/ blends
### Medial
Thanksgiving
harvest

### Blends
leaves

# Vocabulary Pictures

Instructions: _____
_____

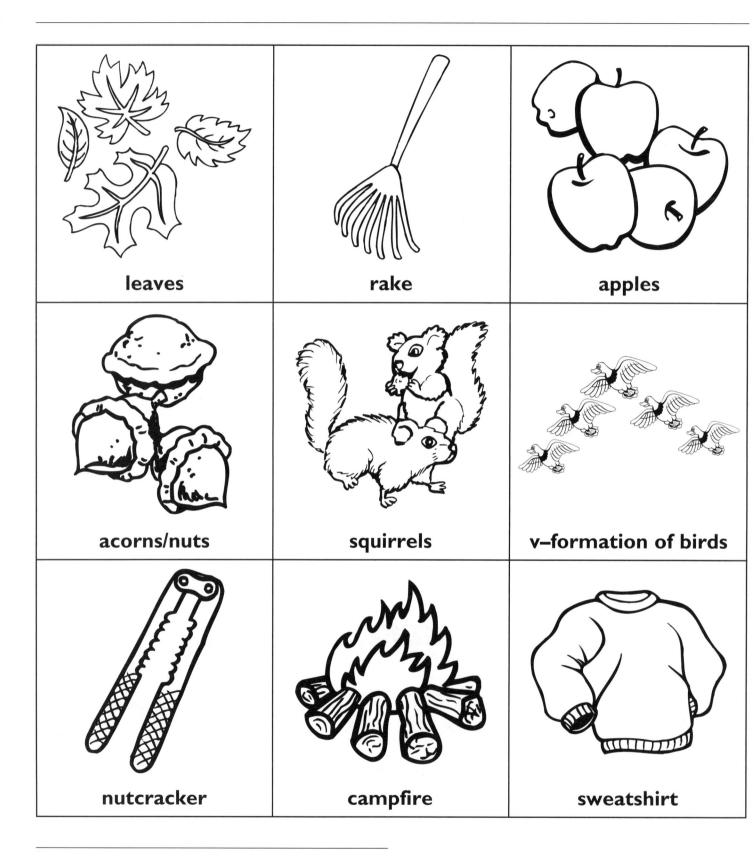

| | | |
|---|---|---|
| **leaves** | **rake** | **apples** |
| **acorns/nuts** | **squirrels** | **v–formation of birds** |
| **nutcracker** | **campfire** | **sweatshirt** |

_____

Name _____ Date _____

Speech-Language Pathologist                    Helper's Signature

#BK-272  Year-Round Literature  •  ©1999 Super Duper® Publications  •  1-800-277-8737  •  www.superduperinc.com

# Vocabulary Pictures

**Instructions:** _____

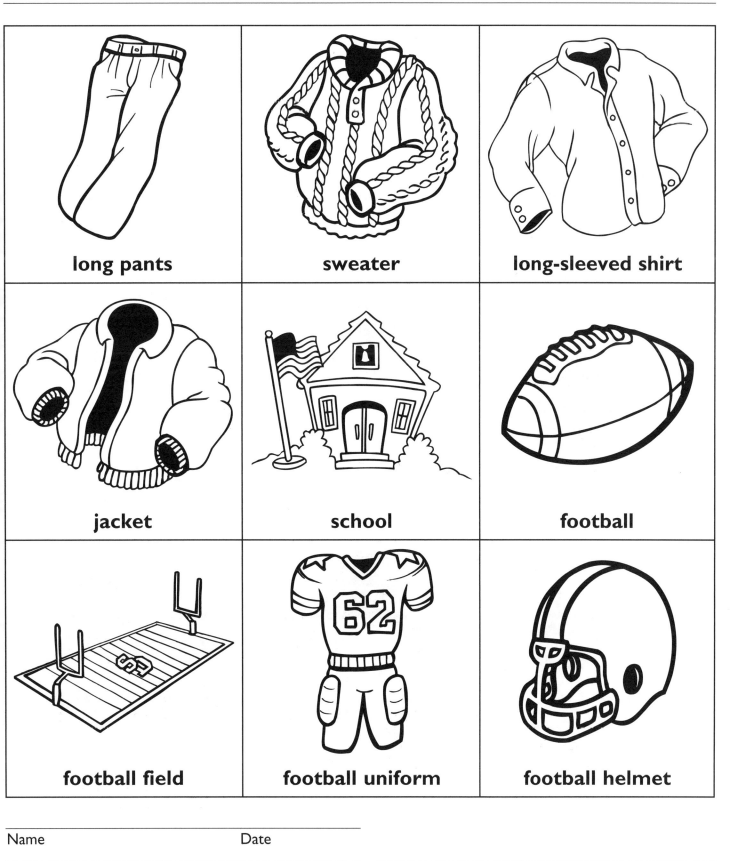

| long pants | sweater | long-sleeved shirt |
| jacket | school | football |
| football field | football uniform | football helmet |

Name _____    Date _____

# Vocabulary Pictures

**Instructions:** _____

_____

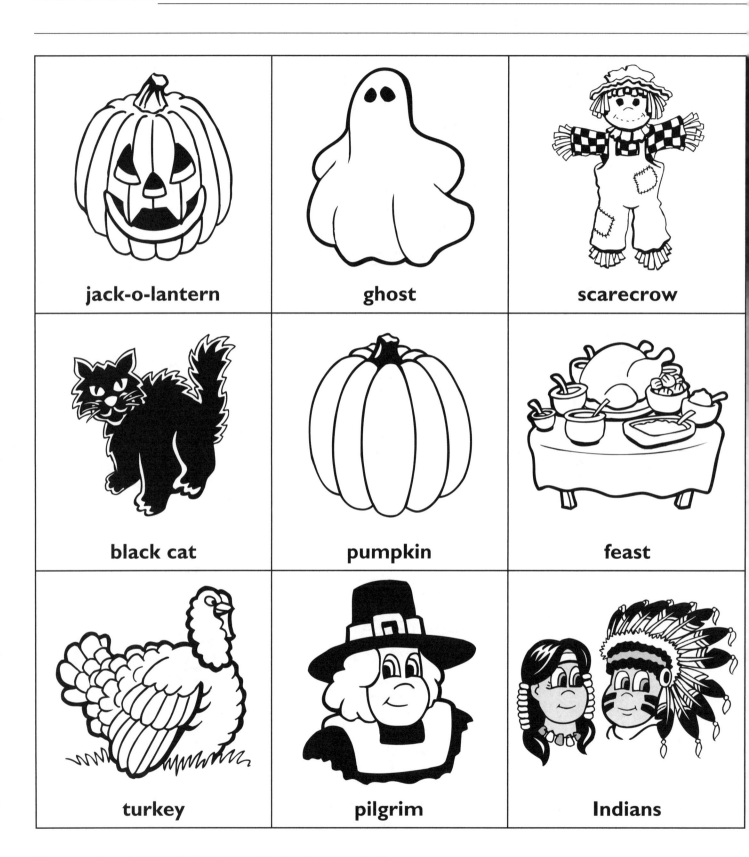

| | | |
|---|---|---|
| jack-o-lantern | ghost | scarecrow |
| black cat | pumpkin | feast |
| turkey | pilgrim | Indians |

Name _____ Date _____

_____

Speech-Language Pathologist      Helper's Signature

#BK-272  Year-Round Literature  •  ©1999 Super Duper® Publications  •  1-800-277-8737  •  www.superduperinc.com

# Story Pattern

**Name:** _____

_____

_____

_____

_____

_____

_____

_____

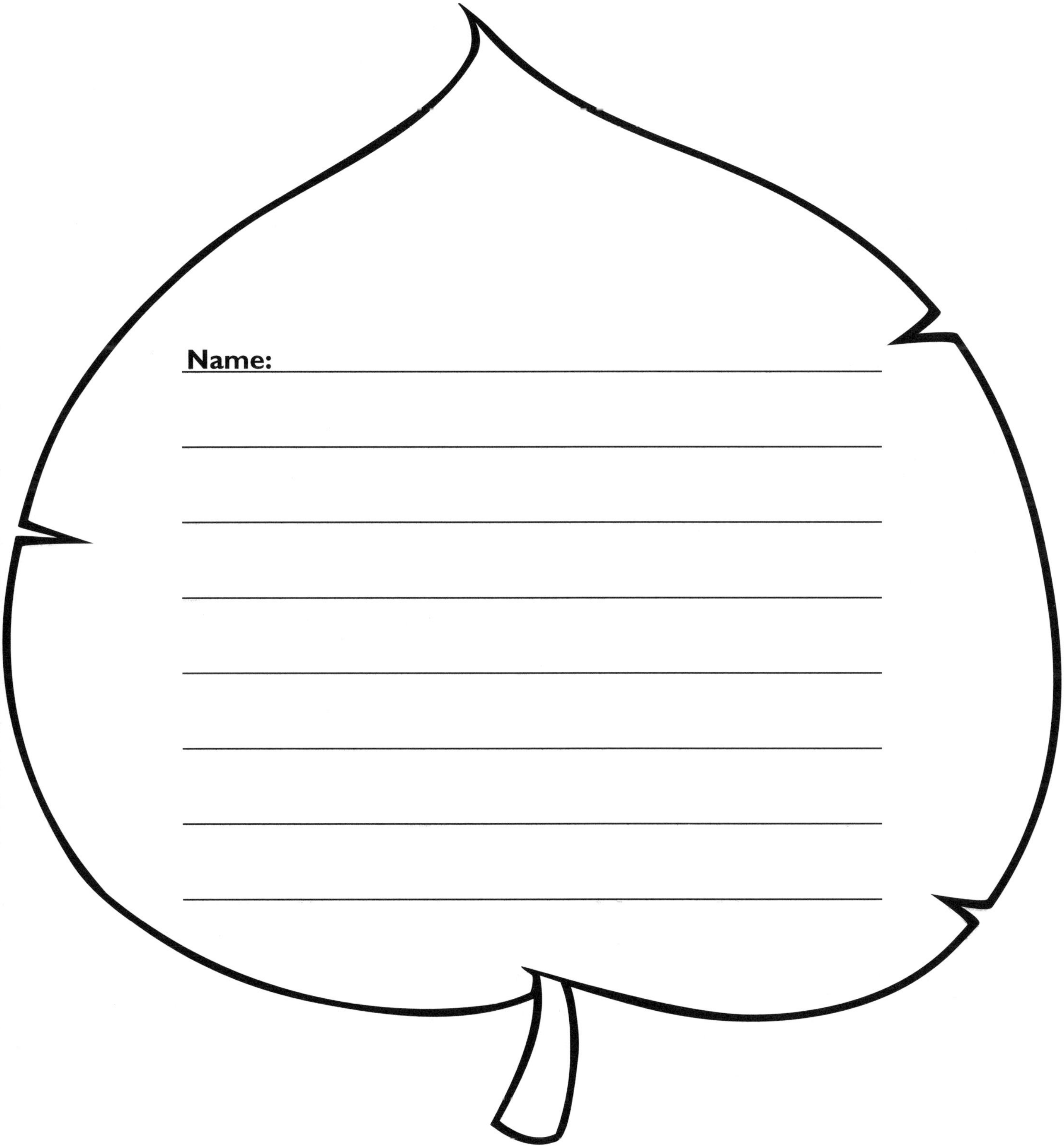

_____
Name

_____
Date

_____
Speech-Language Pathologist

_____
Helper's Signature

#BK-272  Year-Round Literature  •  ©1999 Super Duper® Publications  •  1-800-277-8737  •  www.superduperinc.com

# Red Leaf, Yellow Leaf
## by Lois Ehlert

This is a story about a child going with his dad to pick up a sugar maple tree from the garden center. They take the tree home and plant it in the ground. The story describes the sugar maple tree in the different seasons. The child's favorite time to see the sugar maple tree is in the fall because of the beautifully colored leaves.

---

**Language Expansion:** The following questions can be used to address students' recall of this book or to expand upon concepts addressed in this book.

## Definition
1. What is a tree?
2. What is a leaf?
3. What is a seedling?
4. What is a garden center?
5. What is a spade?

## Function
1. What are seeds used for?
2. What is a spade used for?
3. What is a hole used for?
4. What are roots used for?
5. What is soil used for?

## Category
1. Name three kinds of trees.
2. Name three colors that leaves change in the fall.
3. Name three things you would find at a garden center.
4. Name three things that you can do with a leaf.
5. Name three parts of a tree.

## Description
1. Tell me three things about a tree.
2. Tell me three things about a seed.
3. Tell me three things about a gardener.
4. Tell me three things about the woods.
5. Tell me three things about the fall.

## Vocabulary
Make a sentence using the following words.
1. seed
2. leaves
3. root
4. sprout
5. trunk

## Rhyming
Name a rhyming word for each word below.
1. spade
2. seed
3. roots
4. tree
5. hole

---

## Sequencing
As your students sequence the events in this story, use this list as a guide.
1. Seeds fall from a maple tree and are covered with snow.
2. The spring sun warms the seeds and they grow into a tree.
3. Nursery workers uproot and replant the tree.
4. A family buys the tree, takes it home, and plants it in their yard.
5. Each season the tree looks different, but the child in the family likes the tree best in the fall because the leaves change from green to red to yellow.

#BK-272 Year-Round Literature • ©1999 Super Duper® Publications • 1-800-277-8737 • www.superduperinc.com

# The Apple Pie Tree
## by Zoe Hall

A girl and her sister have a favorite tree in their yard—an apple tree.  The story follows the apple tree through each season of the year.  In the fall, the apples are ready to be picked and the family makes an apple pie.

**Language Expansion:**  The following questions can be used to address students' recall of this book or to expand upon concepts addressed in this book.

## Definition
1. What are apples?
2. What are robins?
3. What is a nest?
4. What are blossoms?
5. What are branches?

## Function
1. What is a nest used for?
2. What is a basket used for?
3. What are apples used for?
4. What is an oven used for?
5. What is apple pie used for?

## Category
1. Name three parts of a tree.
2. Name three colors of apples.
3. Name three ingredients of an apple pie.
4. Name three foods you can make with apples.
5. Name the four seasons.

## Description
1. Tell me three things about an apple pie.
2. Tell me three things about an apple tree.
3. Tell me three things about a nest.
4. Tell me three things about leaves.
5. Tell me three things about robins.

## Vocabulary
Make a sentence using the following words.
1. apple
2. robin
3. cinnamon
4. oven
5. blossom

## Rhyming
Name a rhyming word for each word below.
1. nest
2. pie
3. fall
4. pick
5. yard

## Sequencing
As your students sequence the events in this story, use this list as a guide.
1. In the winter, the apple tree is brown and bare.
2. In the spring, leaves grow on every branch, blossoms appear, and apples begin to grow.
3. In the summer, the apples get bigger and bigger.
4. In the autumn, the apples are picked.
5. The family makes an apple pie out of the apples from the tree.

# Sun, Snow, Stars and Sky
## by Catherine and Laurence Anholt

This is a wonderful book that addresses each of the four seasons. Each page has illustrations and text that describe the highlights of the season. The book can be used to help the children think and talk about the changing seasons.

**Language Expansion:** The following questions can be used to address students' recall of this book or to expand upon concepts addressed in this book.

## Definition
1. What is the morning?
2. What is hibernating?
3. What is wind?
4. What is a bonfire?
5. What does wet mean?

## Function
1. What is a bonfire used for?
2. What is an umbrella used for?
3. What is a rake used for?
4. What is ice used for?
5. What is a scarf used for?

## Category
1. Name three kinds of warm drinks.
2. Name three kinds of nuts.
3. Name three animals that live where it is cold.
4. Name three things to do in the snow.
5. Name three things that can grow on trees.

## Description
1. Tell me about the weather in the fall.
2. Tell me three things about windy days.
3. Tell me three things about hot days.
4. Tell me three things about cold days.
5. Tell me three things about trees.

## Vocabulary
Make a sentence using the following words.
1. harvest
2. wind
3. puddle
4. glove
5. berries

## Rhyming
Name a rhyming word for each word below.
1. fire
2. wet
3. rake
4. ice
5. snow

## Sequencing
As your students sequence the events in this story, use this list as a guide.
1. The book talks about different kinds of weather.
2. The book talks about hot days.
3. The book talks about cold days.
4. The book talks about the weather in the spring, summer, autumn, and winter.
5. The book talks about how the weather changes each day.

#BK-272 Year-Round Literature • ©1999 Super Duper® Publications • 1-800-277-8737 • www.superduperinc.com

# Fall Articulation and Language Games

(The following games can be used with the articulation and vocabulary word list or the literature language questions.)

## Football Game

Photocopy the football pattern (page 12) on brown construction paper. Write the number "1," "2," or "3" on the back of 20 footballs. Write the number 10 on the remaining footballs. Cut out and laminate the footballs. Place footballs number side down on a table. After a student makes a sentence with a fall word containing his/her sound or answers a fall language question, the student may draw a football. The number on the back is the number of points the student receives on the score sheet for that turn. The student with the most points wins.

### Team Approach

In order to win the game, the team must reach a designated number of points. For example, the team must have 30 points by the end of the class to win.

## Tree/Leaf Matching Game

Photocopy the tree and leaf patterns (pages 13 and 14). Color the trees and leaves, cut them apart and laminate them. Lay the cards facedown and allow each student to turn over two cards. If the cards don't match, the student must choose one of the cards to name and describe using good speech and language and then put both cards facedown. If the cards match, the student must tell about the tree and leaf by naming and describing them using good speech and language. Then, the student may keep the matching pair. Continue taking turns until all the trees and leaves have been matched. The student with the most matches is the winner.

### Team Approach

In order to win the game, the team must be able to match all of the trees and leaves by the end of the therapy session.

## Apple Game

Photocopy one basket/apple pattern (page 15) for each student. Color, cut out, and laminate the apples and basket. Give each student a basket to place on the table. Put all of the apple cards facedown in a pile on the table. After a student makes a sentence with a fall word containing his/her sound or answers a fall language question, the student may choose one card from the pile. If the card shows a whole apple, the student puts it in his/her basket. If the card shows an apple with a bite, the student returns the card to the pile. The student with the most apples at the end is the winner, or each student is a winner if he/she has at least five apples in his/her basket.

### Language Extension

Talk about how apples grow, different types of apples, and what we can do with apples. Taste various types of apples or have a drink of apple cider.

## Pumpkin Pie Game

Photocopy the pumpkin pie pattern (page 16) for each student. Color, laminate, and cut out the pieces of the pie. Turn the pieces over and place them in a pile on the table. After a student makes a sentence with a fall word containing his/her sound or answers a fall language question, he/she may turn over one piece of pie. In order to win the game, each student must have a whole pie by the end of the class.

### Language Extension

Bring in a recipe book and find recipes for pies. Talk about the different ingredients and steps for making a pie.

## Rake Up Game

Photocopy, color, and laminate the leaf pattern (page 17). Turn the leaves facedown. After a student makes a sentence with a fall word containing his/her sound or answers a fall language question, the student chooses one leaf card. If the leaf has directions, the student must follow the directions. If the leaf is blank, the student may keep the leaf. The student with the most leaves at the end of the game is the winner.

### Team Approach

In order to win the game, the team must get a designated number of leaves. For example, the team must have 15 leaves by the end of the class to win.

# Football Game

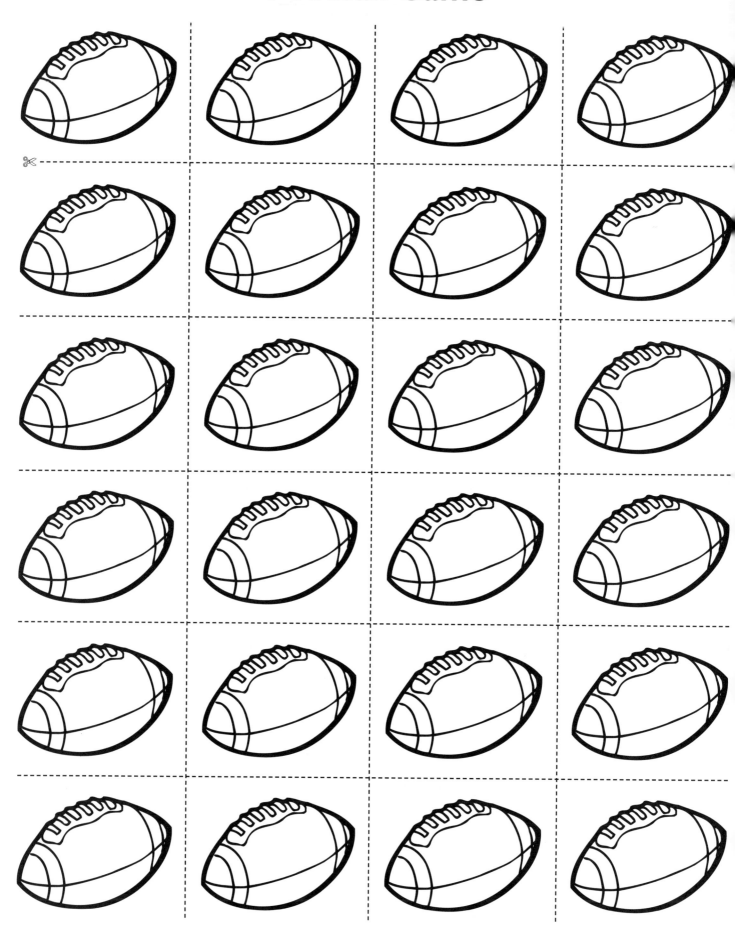

#BK-272  Year-Round Literature  •  ©1999 Super Duper® Publications  •  1-800-277-8737  •  www.superduperinc.com

# Tree/Leaf Matching Game

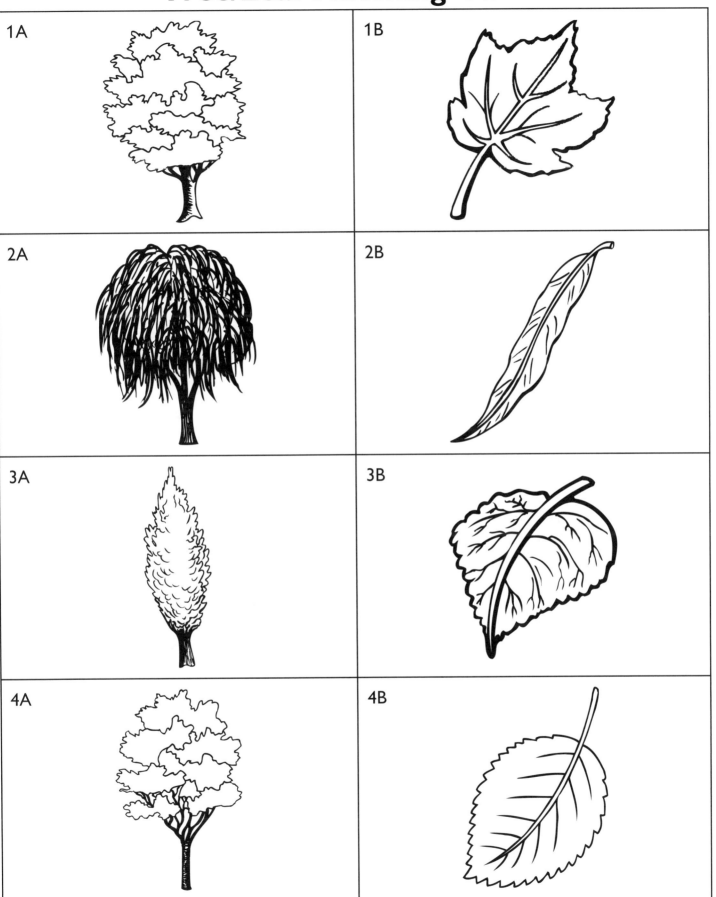

1A

1B

2A

2B

3A

3B

4A

4B

Answers: 1. maple tree/leaf; 2. willow tree/leaf; 3. poplar tree/leaf; 4. birch tree/leaf

# Tree/Leaf Matching Game

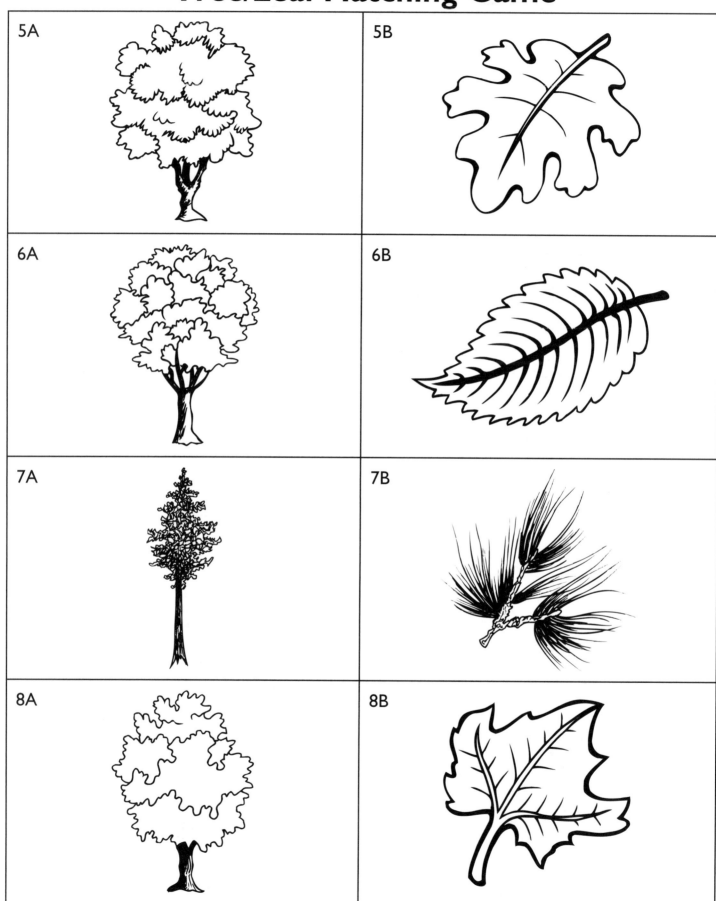

5A

5B

6A

6B

7A

7B

8A

8B

Answers: 5. oak tree/leaf; 6. elm tree/leaf; 7. pine tree/leaf; 8. sycamore tree/leaf

#BK-272 Year-Round Literature • ©1999 Super Duper® Publications • 1-800-277-8737 • www.superduperinc.com

# Apple Game

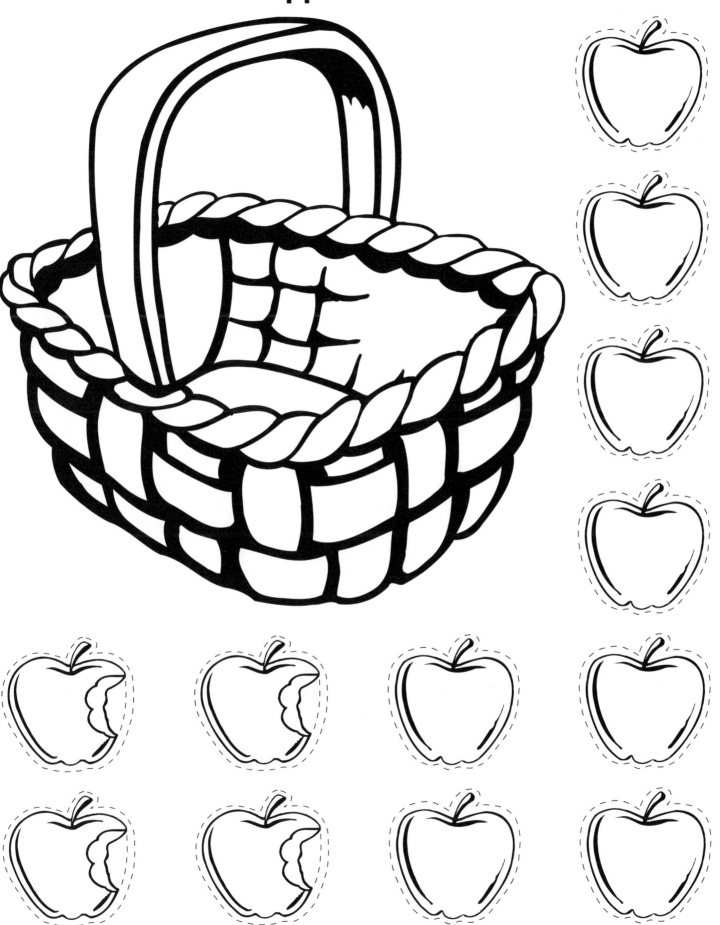

# Pumpkin Pie Game

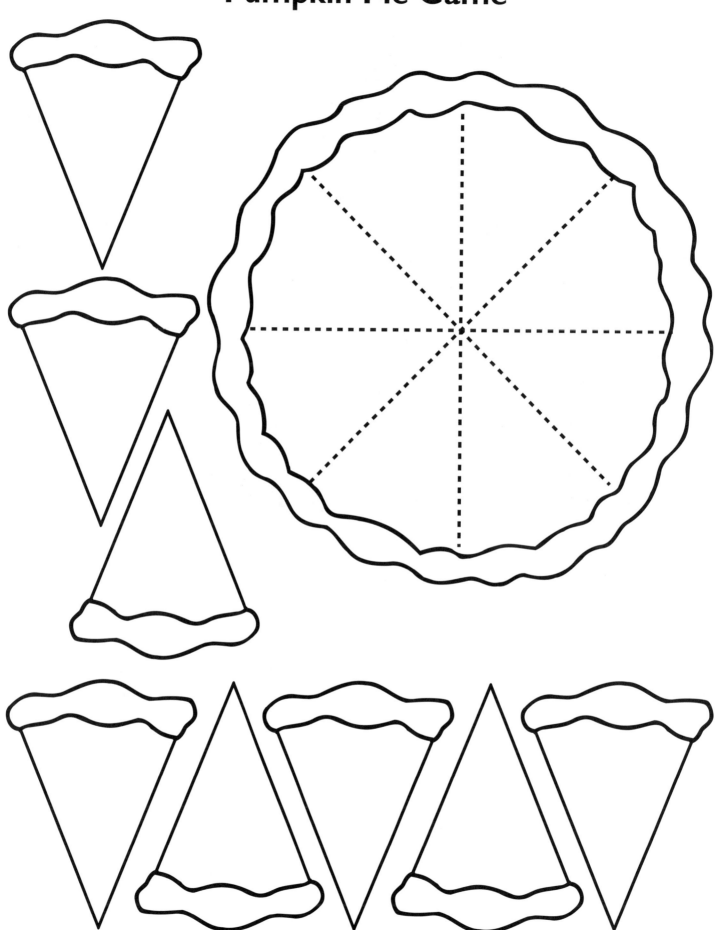

#BK-272  Year-Round Literature  •  ©1999 Super Duper® Publications  •  1-800-277-8737  •  www.superduperinc.com

# Rake Up Game

**Wind blows. Lose leaf**

**It starts to rain. Put 2 leaves back.**

**Bought a new rake. Choose 1 leaf.**

**A friend comes to help. Choose 2 leaves.**

**Wow! What a pile! Choose 3 leaves.**

**It's great for kite flying. Choose 2 leaves.**

# A Bushel of Good Speech

Write words with the _____ sound on each apple. Then, make a sentence with each word out loud using your good speech.

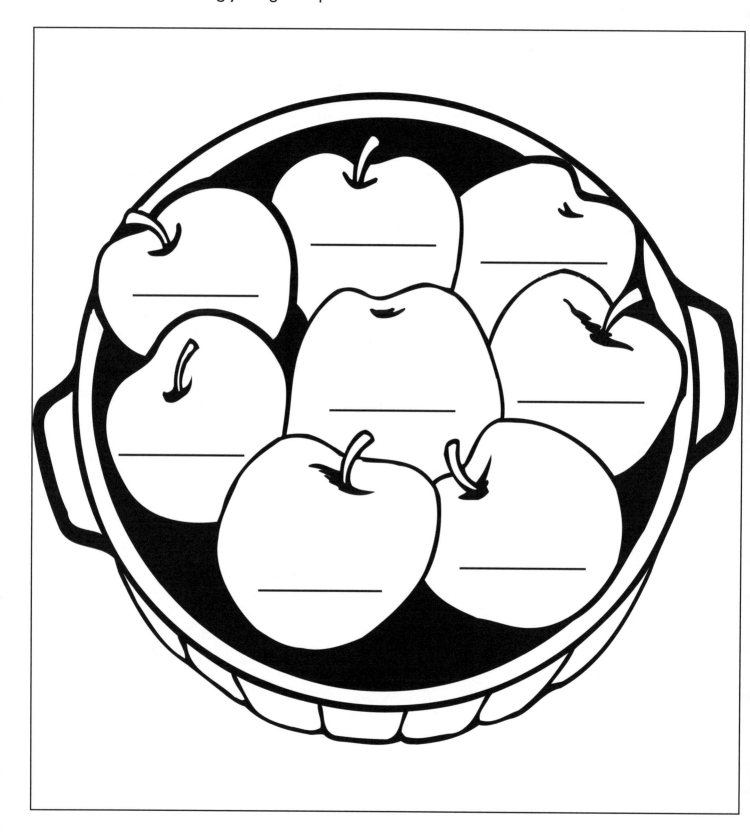

Name _____   Date _____

Speech-Language Pathologist _____   Helper's Signature

# Fall Clothing Hidden Pictures

In the fall when the weather is cooler, you need to wear warmer clothing. Circle the clothing items that you might wear in the fall. Then, tell about each picture using your good speech.

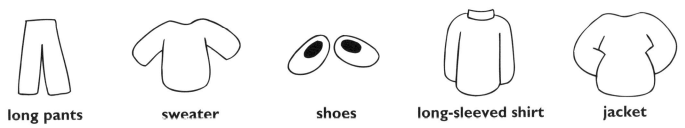

long pants        sweater        shoes        long-sleeved shirt        jacket

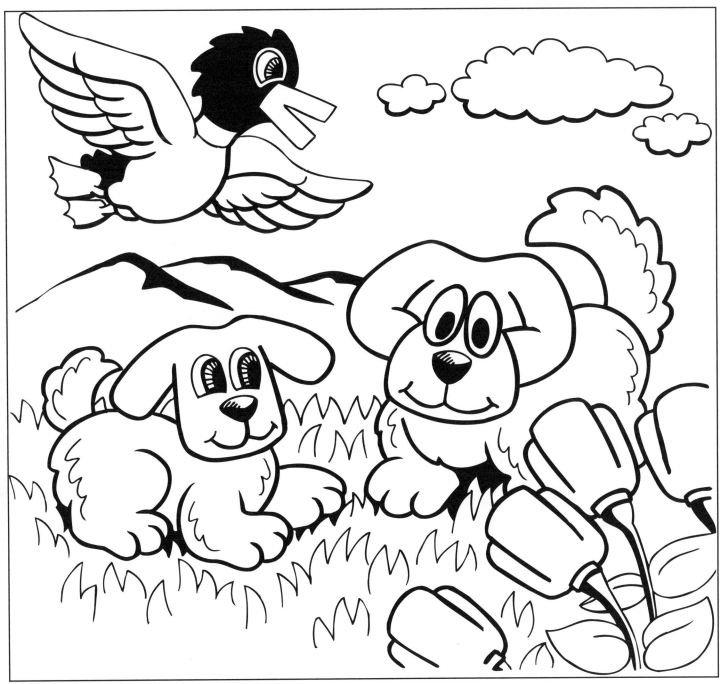

Name _____        Date _____

_____

Speech-Language Pathologist

Helper's Signature _____

#BK-272 Year-Round Literature • ©1999 Super Duper® Publications • 1-800-277-8737 • www.superduperinc.com

# Fall Fun

Tell what is happening in each fall picture below. Which picture do you think shows the most fun? Why? Tell three things that you like about fall.

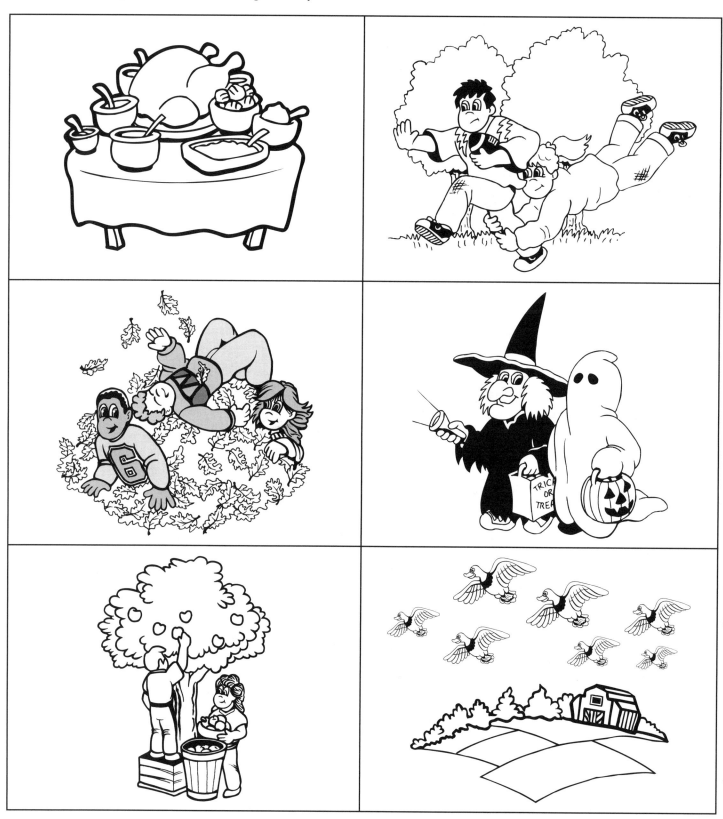

Name _____   Date _____

#BK-272  Year-Round Literature  •  ©1999 Super Duper® Publications  •  1-800-277-8737  •  www.superduperinc.com

# Winter

# Winter Articulation & Vocabulary Word Lists

These word lists are a good resource for articulation and/or vocabulary building activities.

## /r/ and /r/ blends

### Initial
ribbon
red
Rudolph
Red-Nosed

### Medial
fireplace
earmuffs
garland
Silver Bells
January
February
hibernation
Martin Luther King, Jr.

### Final
winter
December
fire
New Year
heater

### Blends
frosty
Christmas Tree
presents
evergreen tree
Groundhog Day
frostbite
Christmas
freeze
snowdrift
green
wreath
scarf
ornaments
cards
hearth
March
short days
blizzard
Valentine's Heart

## /s/ amd /s/ blend

### Initial
season
Silver Bells
Silent Night
Santa Claus

### Medial
presents
December
icicles
ice hockey
poinsettia

### Final
earmuffs
ornaments
ice
fireplace

### Blends
scarf
snow
snowballs
snowman
snow angel
snow fort
snowsuit
sled
stockings
ski
sled
snowdrift
snow plow
snow shovel
snowflake
snowstorm
sleigh
Washington
frosty
Christmas
Christmas Tree
ice skate
frostbite

## /z/

### Medial
presents
blizzard
Valentine's Day

### Final
gloves
mittens
long johns
Jingle Bells
cards
bells
short days
freeze
New Year's
Santa Claus
Silver Bells
snowballs
stockings

## /l/ and /l/ blends

### Initial
long johns
long pants
Lincoln

### Medial
hot chocolate
holly
Silent Night
holiday
Valentine's Day
garland
Valentine's Heart

### Final
snowball

### Blends
gloves
sled
Santa Claus
blizzard

igloo
sleigh
blanket
Jingle Bells
Silver Bells
candles
icicles
fireplace
snowflake
igloo
sleigh
shovel
angel

## /k/ and /k/ blends
cold
cards
candles
coat

### Medial
hot chocolate
Hanukkah
stockings
hockey
hockey puck
hockey stick

### Final
snowflake
puck
stick

### Blends
scarf
Santa Claus
ice skating
clover

 #BK-272  Year-Round Literature • ©1999 Super Duper® Publications • 1-800-277-8737 • www.superduperinc.com

# Winter Articulation & Vocabulary Word Lists (Cont.)

## /g/ and /g/ blends
### Initial
garland

### Blends
gloves
Groundhog Day
evergreen tree
igloo

## /th/
### Initial
thermometer
thaw
thermal underwear

### Medial
cold weather
winter clothing
Martin Luther King, Jr.

### Final
wreath
hearth

## /sh/
### Initial
short days
shiver

### Medial
snow shovel
Washington
snowshoes

### Final
slush

## /ch/
### Initial
chimney
chill
chilly
chipmunk

### Medial
hot chocolate
wind chill

### Final
March

## /m/ and /m/ blends
### Initial
mittens
March
melt
Martin Luther King, Jr.

### Medial
snowman
Christmas
ornaments
earmuffs
snowmobile

### Blends
December

## /p/ and /p/ blends
### Initial
poinsettia

### Medial
ski pole
hockey puck

### Blends
presents
snowplow
fireplace

## /b/ and /b/ blends
### Initial
bells
boots

### Medial
snowballs

ribbon
February
hibernation
frostbite
toboggan

### Blends
blizzard
December

## /f/ and /f/ blends
### Initial
February
fire
fireplace

### Medial
ice fishing

### Final
scarf
earmuff

### Blends
frosty
frozen
freeze
frostbite
snowdrift

## /v/ and /v/ blends
### Initial
Valentine's Heart

### Final
bear cave

### Blends
gloves
snow shovel
scarves

# Vocabulary Pictures

**Instructions:** _____

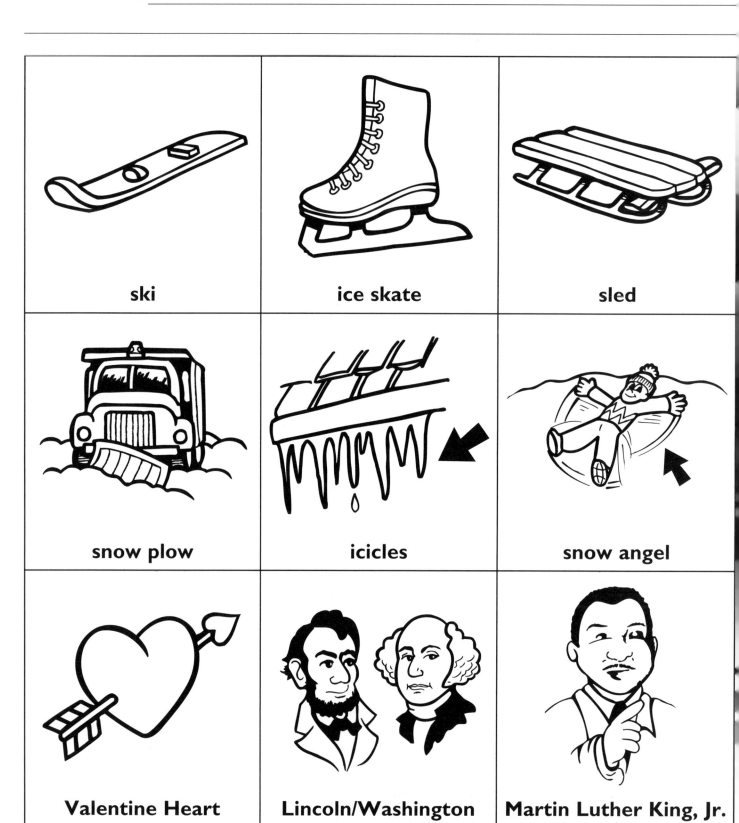

ski

ice skate

sled

snow plow

icicles

snow angel

**Valentine Heart**

**Lincoln/Washington**

**Martin Luther King, Jr.**

Name

Date

Speech-Language Pathologist

Helper's Signature

#BK-272  Year-Round Literature • ©1999 Super Duper® Publications • 1-800-277-8737 • www.superduperinc.com

# Vocabulary Pictures

**Instructions:** _____

_____

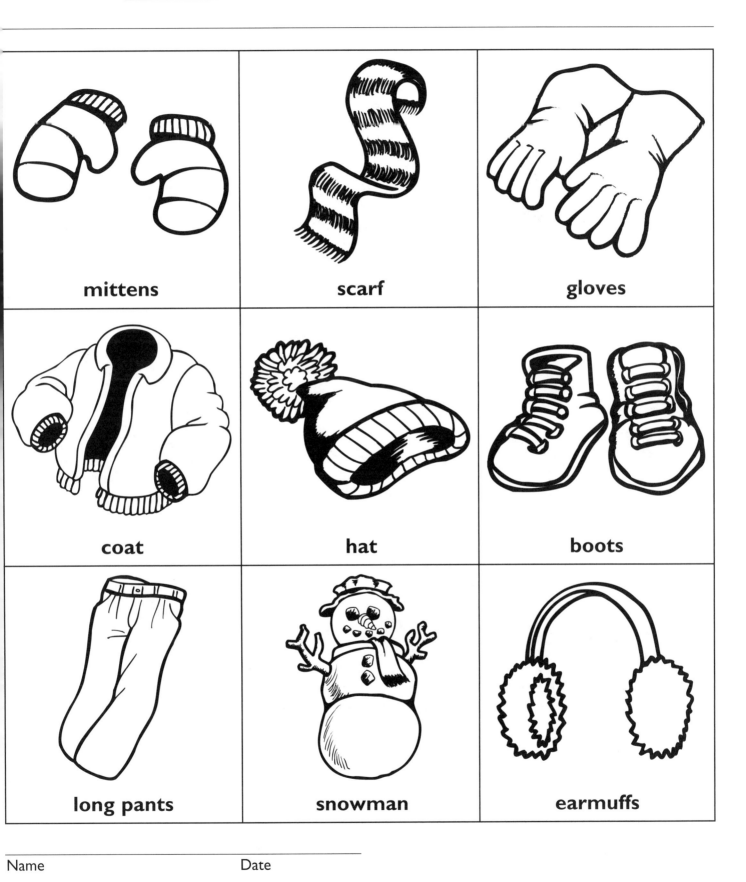

| | | |
|---|---|---|
| mittens | scarf | gloves |
| coat | hat | boots |
| long pants | snowman | earmuffs |

Name _____   Date _____

Speech-Language Pathologist              Helper's Signature

# Vocabulary Pictures

**Instructions:** _____

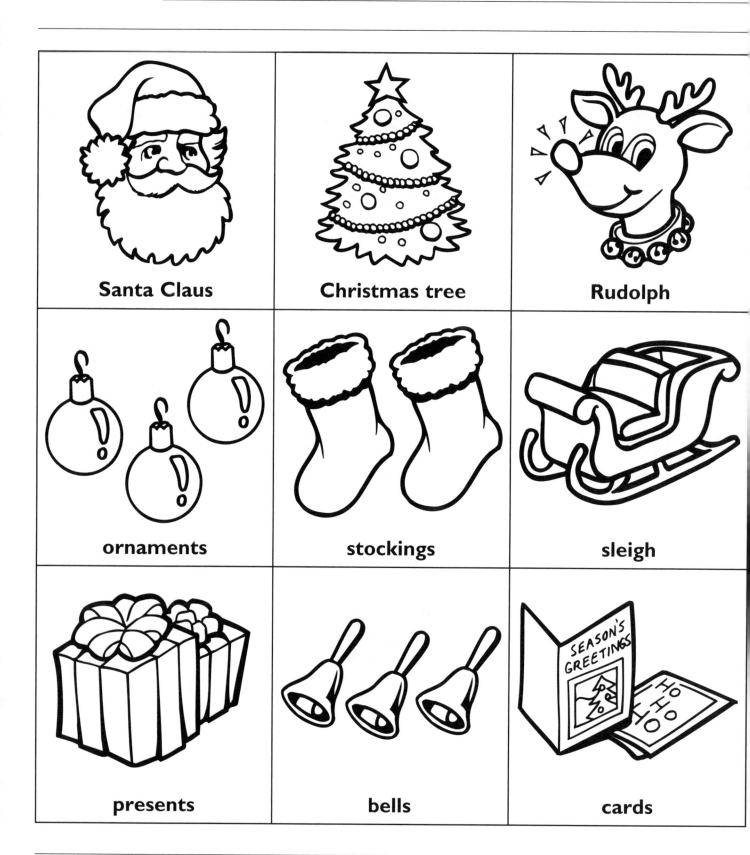

| | | |
|---|---|---|
| **Santa Claus** | **Christmas tree** | **Rudolph** |
| ornaments | stockings | sleigh |
| presents | bells | cards |

Name _____     Date _____

Speech-Language Pathologist          Helper's Signature

#BK-272  Year-Round Literature  •  ©1999 Super Duper® Publications  •  1-800-277-8737  •  www.superduperinc.com

# Story Pattern

**Name:** _____

_____

_____

_____

_____

_____

_____

_____

_____

_____

_____

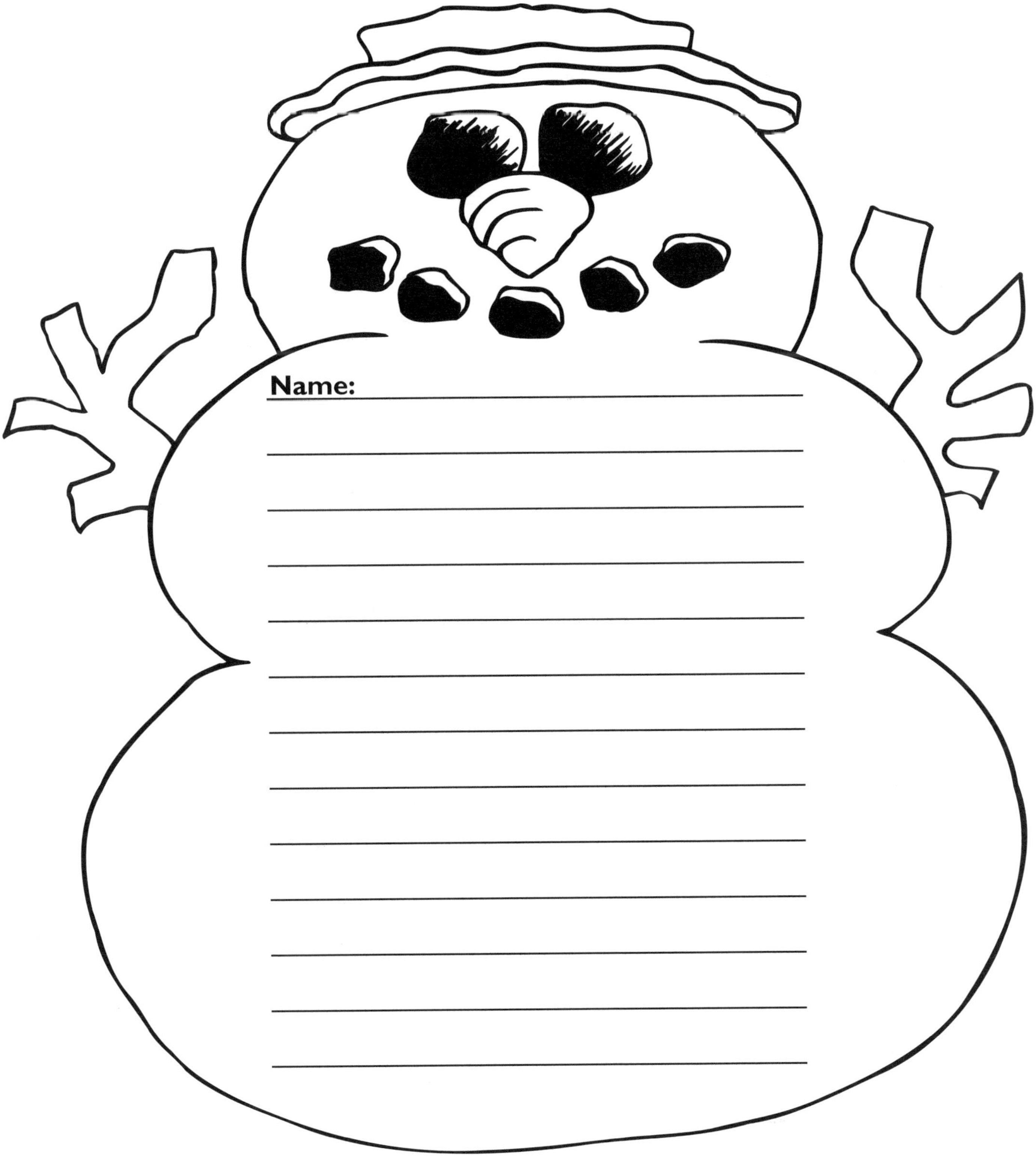

Name _____     Date _____

Speech-Language Pathologist                    Helper's Signature

# The Mitten
## by Jan Brett

This is a Ukrainian folk tale about a little boy who had white mittens. While playing in the snow, he lost one of his mittens. The story tells about all the animals that get inside of the mitten to stay warm. Finally, the last of the animals gets in and sneezes. They all fall out of the mitten and it shoots up into the air. The little boy sees his lost mitten fly into the air and is so happy to find it.

**Language Expansion:** The following questions can be used to address students' recall of this book or to expand upon concepts addressed in this book.

## Definition
1. What are mittens?
2. What is wool?
3. What is knitting?
4. What is cozy?
5. What is a sneeze?

## Function
1. What is wool used for?
2. What is a mitten used for?
3. What is snow used for?
4. What is a fireplace used for?
5. What is a hat used for?

## Category
1. Name three things you can make with wool.
2. Name three things Nicki wore to keep warm.
3. Name three colors that could be used to make mittens.
4. Name three animals that go into Nicki's mitten.
5. Name three things that you can do with winter snow.

## Description
1. Tell me three things about winter.
2. Tell me three things about snow.
3. Tell me three things about mittens.
4. Tell me three things about the bear.
5. Tell me three things about the mouse.

## Vocabulary
Make a sentence using the following words.
1. mittens
2. wool
3. knit
4. cozy
5. sneeze

## Rhyming
Name a rhyming word for each word below.
1. wool
2. sneeze
3. hat
4. bear
5. knit

## Sequencing
As your students sequence the events in this story, use this list as a guide.
1. Nicki wants mittens made from wool white as snow.
2. His grandmother thinks it is not the best idea because Nicki might lose them in the snow, but she finally makes them for Nicki.
3. Nicki loses a mitten in the snow.
4. Several animals try to fit in the warm mitten, but the bear sneezes, the animals fall out, and the mitten flies up in the air.
5. Nicki sees the mitten fly up in the air and is so glad to see that he has found his lost mitten.

#BK-272 Year-Round Literature • ©1999 Super Duper® Publications • 1-800-277-8737 • www.superduperinc.com

# Snowballs
## by Lois Ehlert

This is a book about building a family of snow people in the winter. Various items, such as seeds, nuts, yarn, and ethnic clothing, are used to decorate each snow person. The illustrations are quite colorful and appealing to children.

**Language Expansion:** The following questions can be used to address students' recall of this book or to expand upon concepts addressed in this book.

## Definition
1. What is snow?
2. What are seeds?
3. What is a snowman?
4. What is a puddle?
5. What does melting mean?

## Category
1. Name three things you can make with snow.
2. Name three things you can use to decorate a snowman.
3. Name three things that were used to make eyes for the snow people.
4. Name three things that were used to make mouths for the snow people.
5. Name three things that the snow people turned into when the sun came out.

## Vocabulary
Make a sentence using the following words.
1. snow
2. snowball
3. shrinking
4. slush
5. melting

## Function
1. What is snow used for?
2. What is a sock used for?
3. What is a snowball used for?
4. What is a hat used for?
5. What is the sun used for?

## Description
1. Tell me three things about winter.
2. Tell me three things about snow.
3. Tell me three things about making a snowman.
4. Tell me three things about the snow boy.
5. Tell me three things about the snow baby.

## Rhyming
Name a rhyming word for each word below.
1. melt
2. sock
3. sun
4. slush
5. shrink

## Sequencing
As your students sequence the events in this story, use this list as a guide.
1. After it snows, some children make a snow dad and a snow mom.
2. The children make a snow boy.
3. The children make a snow girl.
4. The children make a snow cat and a snow dog.
5. When the sun comes out, the snow family begins to melt.

# The Snowy Day
## by Ezra Keats

This book is about a boy who wakes up and discovers it snowed during the night. The boy walks around the city making footprints, snow angels, and snow balls. This is a delightful book about the winter season.

**Language Expansion:** The following questions can be used to address students' recall of this book or to expand upon concepts addressed in this book.

## Definition
1. What is winter?
2. What is snow?
3. What is a snowsuit?
4. What is a snowman?
5. What is a snow angel?

## Function
1. What is snow used for?
2. What is a snowsuit used for?
3. What is a snowball used for?
4. What is a path used for?
5. What is a pocket used for?

## Category
1. Name three things you can make with snow.
2. Name three things Peter did in the snow.
3. Name three things you wear to stay warm in the snow.
4. Name three things that you can use to decorate a snowman.
5. Name three things that you can put in your pocket.

## Description
1. Tell me three things about winter.
2. Tell me three things about snow.
3. Tell me three things about making a snowman.
4. Tell me three things about a snow angel.
5. Tell me three things about having a snowball fight.

## Vocabulary
Make a sentence using the following words.
1. snow
2. snowsuit
3. tracks
4. snowman
5. melt

## Rhyming
Name a rhyming word for each word below.
1. path
2. pocket
3. tracks
4. night
5. boy

## Sequencing
As your students sequence the events in this story, use this list as a guide.
1. Peter wakes up to a snowy day.
2. Peter goes outside and plays in the snow.
3. Peter makes a snowball and takes it inside.
4. Peter gets ready for bed and his snowball melts.
5. Peter wakes up and more snow is falling so he goes outside with a friend to play again.

#BK-272 Year-Round Literature • ©1999 Super Duper® Publications • 1-800-277-8737 • www.superduperinc.com

# Winter Articulation and Language Games

(The following games can be used with the articulation and vocabulary word list or the literature language questions.)

## Winter Clothing Game

Photocopy the winter clothing pattern (page 32) for each student. Color, cut out, and laminate each winter clothing item. Put the cards in a stocking cap. After a student makes a sentence with a winter word containing his/her sound or answers a winter language question, the student may draw a card from the hat. The object is for each student to get the entire winter outfit by the end of the session.

### Language Extension

After completing the winter outfit, have each student describe each part and tell what each part is used for. Talk about how winter weather varies from place to place and ask the students what someone might wear during the winter season in Hawaii.

### Team Approach

In order to win the game, each team member must complete an entire winter outfit by the end of class.

## Snowflake Game

Photocopy the snowflake pattern (page 33). Cut out and laminate the snowflakes. Place all cards number side down. After a student makes a sentence with a winter word containing his/her sound or answers a winter language question, the student may draw a snowflake. The number on the card is the number of points the student receives on the score sheet for the turn. The student with the most points wins.

### Team Approach

In order to win the game, the team must earn a designated number of points. For example, the team must have 30 points by the end of class to win.

## Snowman Game

Photocopy, color, and laminate the snowman game board (page 35). Copy the student sheet (page 34) for each student. (You can photocopy front and back to save paper and use the back side with the next therapy group.) Make a game die using a penny. Put a piece of masking tape on both sides and write a "2" on one side and a "3" on the other side with permanent ink.

Discuss the different parts of the snowman shown on the game board and tell the class that the goal is for each student to get each part to complete the snowman on the student sheet. Then, give each student a student sheet and pencil. After a student makes a sentence with a winter word containing his/her sound or answers a winter language question, the student may flip the penny die, move the allotted spaces, and then draw the snowman part on the student sheet.

### Language Extension

After completing the snowman, ask the student to talk about other things that can be made from snow. Talk about how snow is made and what happens to snow when the sun comes out.

## Winter Suitcase Game

Gather several winter clothing items and put them in a suitcase or photocopy and cut out the winter suitcase pattern (page 36). Take the suitcase into class and tell the students you have packed for a pretend trip to go skiing in the mountains. Allow the class a few minutes to brainstorm about what's inside the suitcase. (While each student is talking, monitor and correct any target sound production.) Give each student a turn to close his/her eyes and pull an item out of the suitcase. Then, the students must say three sentences about the object using correct speech and language. Continue the game until all of the items have been taken out of the suitcase.

### Language Extension

Ask each student to describe, categorize, and tell the function of each item. Spend time asking "wh" questions such as: "Why would you want to take this object on your ski trip?" or " Where could you find this object?"

## Snowball Fight Game

Make two copies of the snowball pattern (page 37). Cut out and laminate the snowballs. Turn the snowballs upside down and put them in a pile on the table. After a student makes a sentence with his/her sound, or answers a winter language question, the student may turn over one snowball. If the snowball says "Hit," the student keeps it. If it says "Miss," the student puts it back. The one with the most snowballs at the end of the class wins.

### Team Approach

In order to win, the team must earn a designated number of snowballs. For example, the team must have 15 snowballs by the end of the class to win.

# Winter Clothing Game

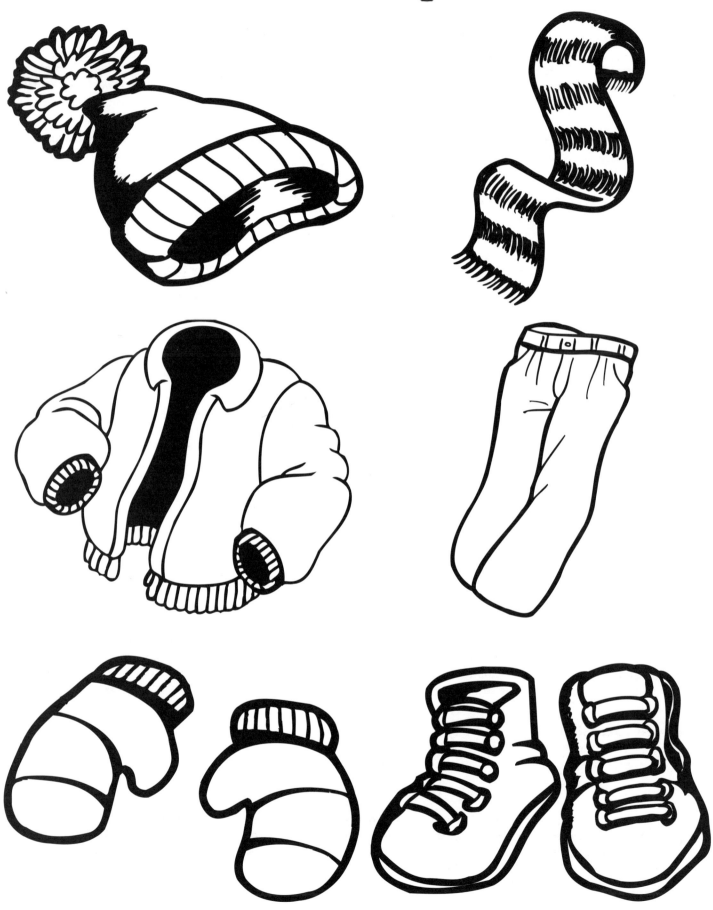

 #BK-272  Year-Round Literature  •  ©1999 Super Duper® Publications  •  1-800-277-8737  •  www.superduperinc.com

# Snowflake Game

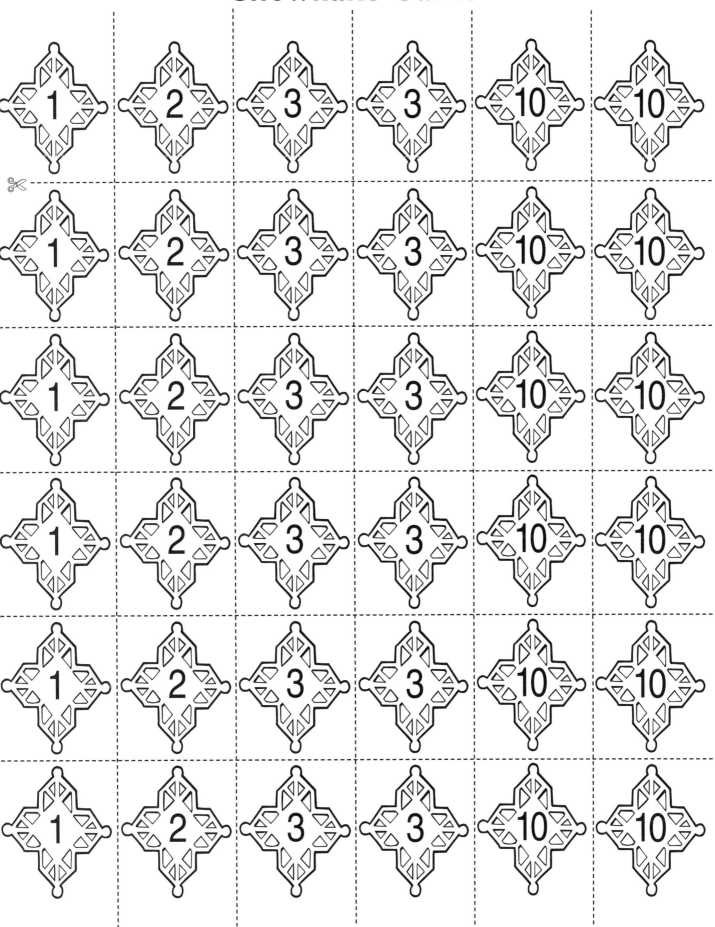

# Snowman Game Student Sheet

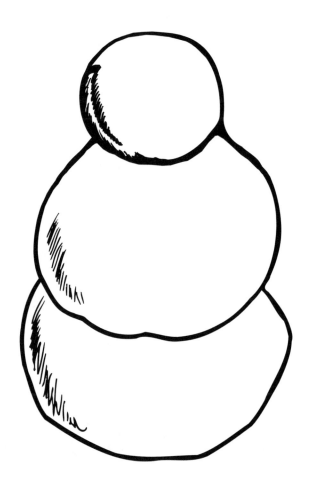

# Snowman Game Board

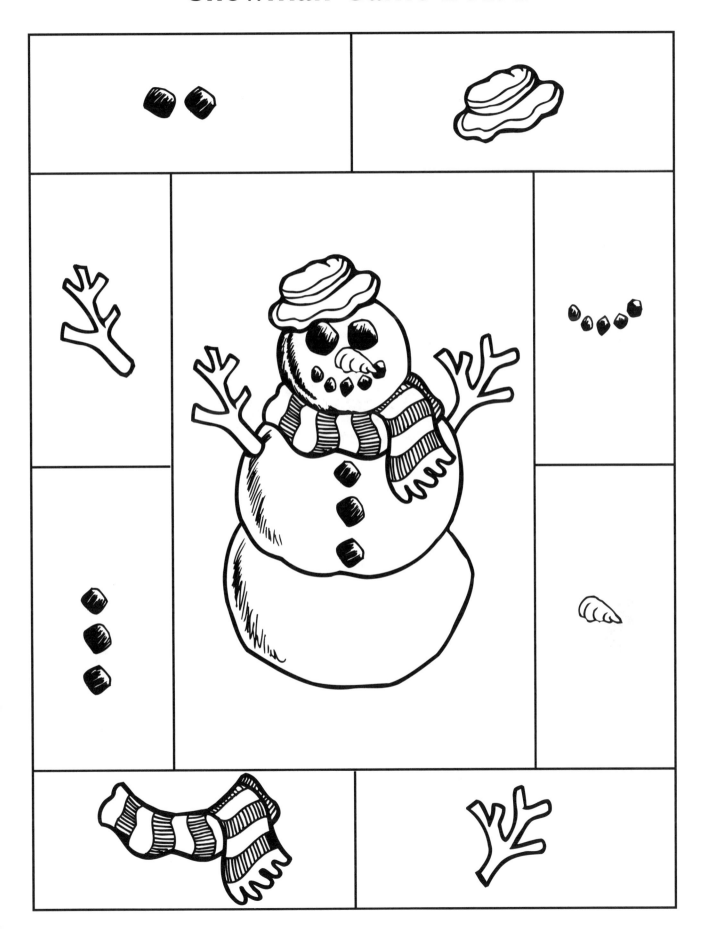

# Winter Suitcase Game

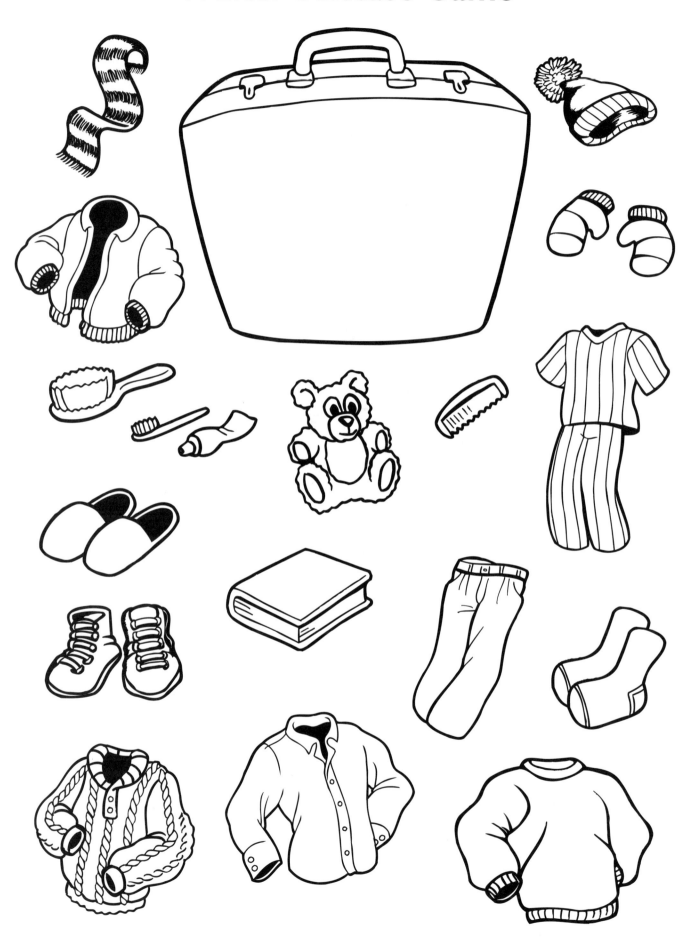

# Snowball Fight Game

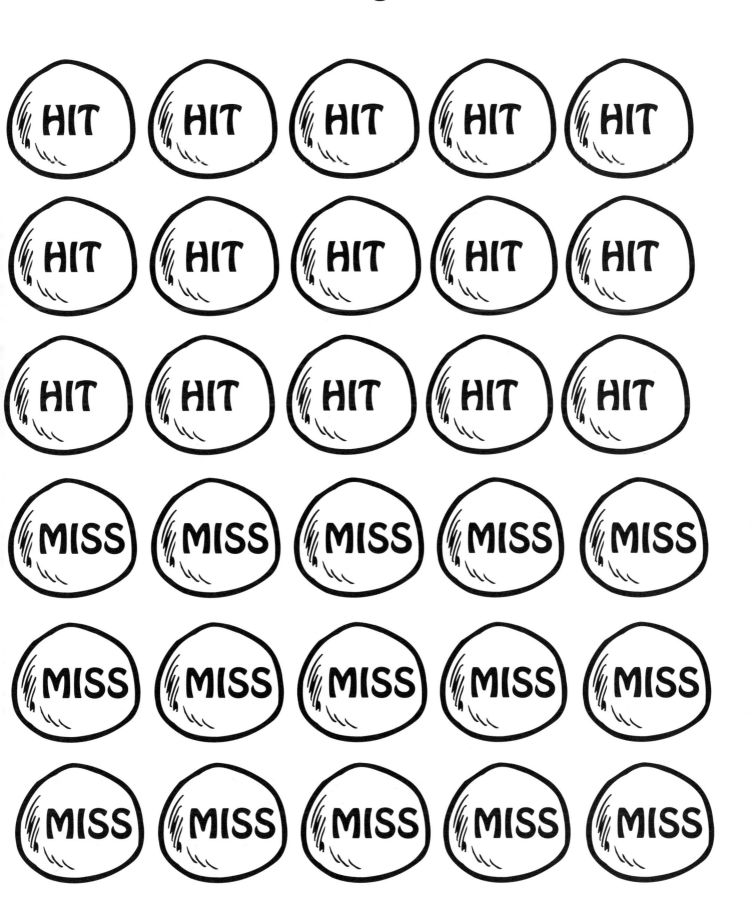

# It's Snowing Good Speech

Write words with the _____ sound on each snowflake. Then, make a sentence with each word out loud using your good speech.

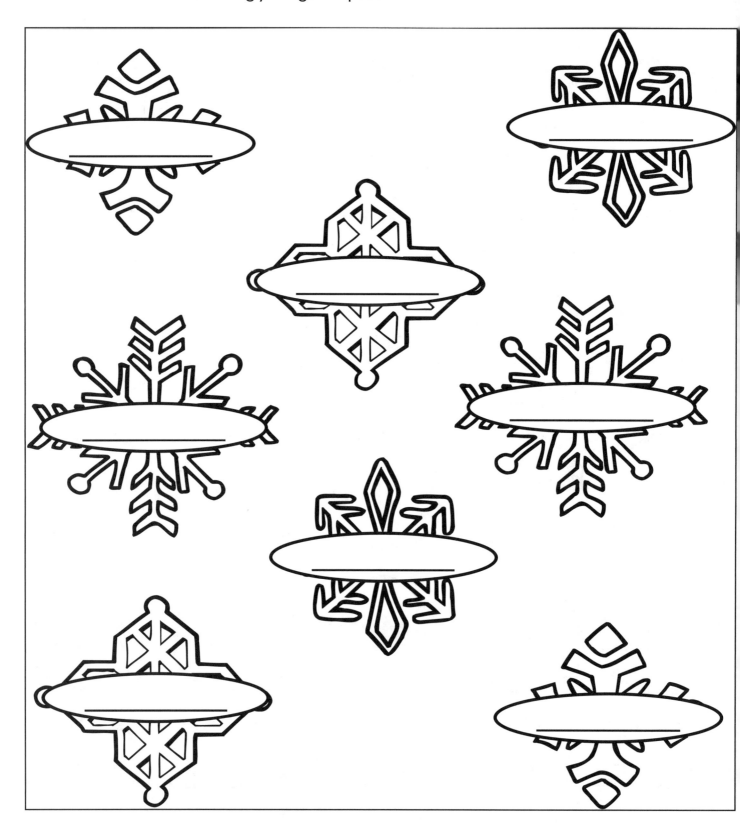

Name _____

Date _____

Speech-Language Pathologist _____

Helper's Signature _____

#BK-272  Year-Round Literature • ©1999 Super Duper® Publications • 1-800-277-8737 • www.superduperinc.com

# Winter Clothing Hidden Pictures

In the winter, when the weather is colder, you need to wear warmer clothing. Circle the clothing items that you might wear in the winter. Then, tell about each picture using your good speech.

**Boots**    **Coat**    **Scarf**    **Earmuffs**    **Mittens**    **Hat**

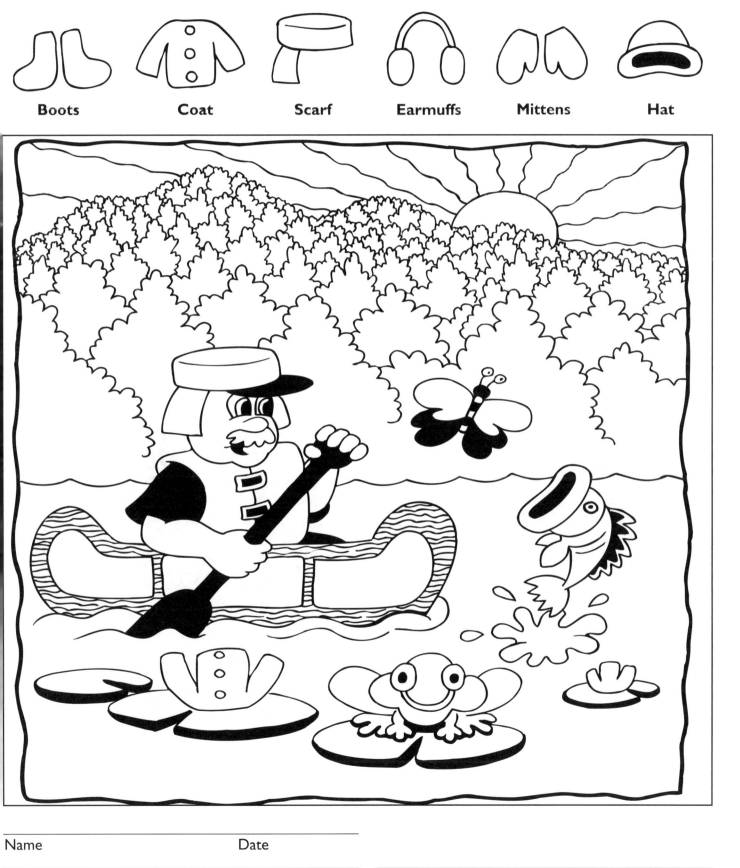

Name _____    Date _____

_____

Speech-Language Pathologist

_____

Helper's Signature

# The Four Seasons

1. What season does each picture show?
2. What season are we in now?

3. What will be our next season?
4. Tell two things about each season using the pictures below

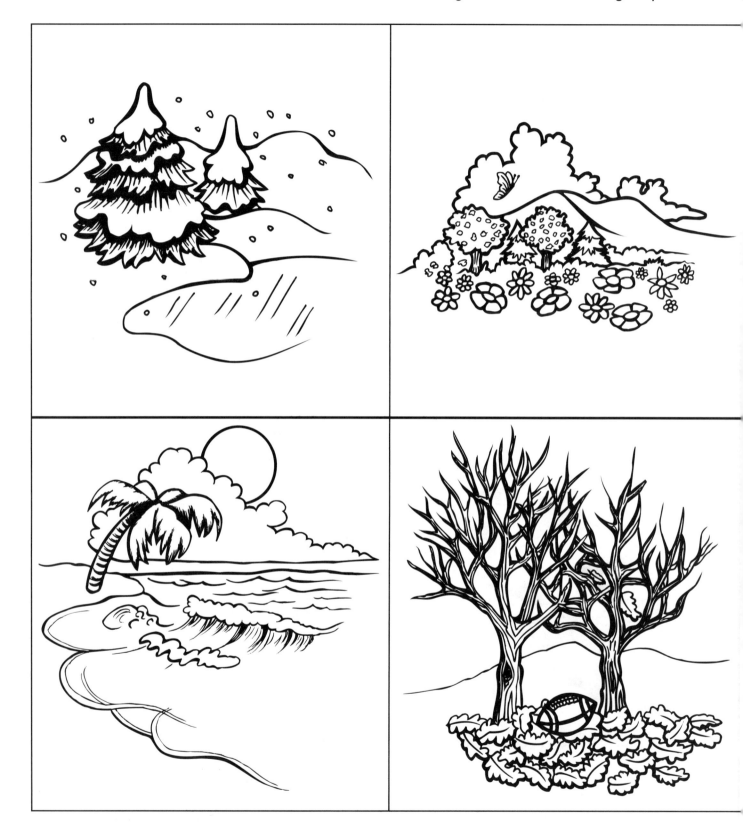

Name _____ Date _____

# Spring

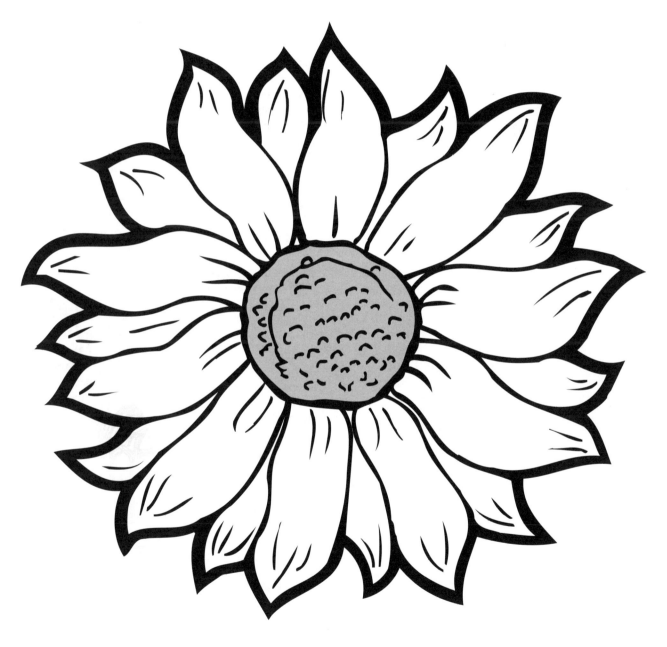

# Spring Articulation & Vocabulary Word Lists

These word lists are a good resource for articulation and/or vocabulary building activities.

## /r/ and /r/ blends

### Initial
rainbow
rake
robin
rose
raincoat

### Medial
carnation
carrot
orchid
iris
flowerpot
marigold
butterfly

### Final
flower
weather
clover
spring fever
fertilizer
water
lawn mower
Easter
sunflower
feather

### Blends
spring
grow
sprout
green grass
drizzle
strawberry
spring break
frog
umbrella
snapdragon
branch
breeze
tree
garden
short-sleeved shirt
chirp
bluebird
April Fool's Day
dirt
hummingbird
clippers
corn
cardinal

April
March
warm
leprechaun

## /s/ and /s/ blends

### Initial
seeds
sunflower
season
sun
soil
seedling

### Medial
baseball
insects

### Final
rain boots
pants
shorts
lettuce
plants
green grass
iris

### Blends
short-sleeved shirt
sprout
strawberries
spring
snapdragon
nest
Easter bunny
Easter basket
spring cleaning
spring fever
spring break

## /z/

### Initial
zinnia

### Medial
pansy
daisy
drizzle
fertilizer
### Final

eggs
seeds
leaves
rose
clippers
green beans
flowers
baby animals
daffodils
worms
hose
buds
weeds
tadpoles
eggshells
blossoms
feathers
breeze
petals
frogs
bees
Easter eggs
wildflowers

## /l/ and /l/ blends

### Initial
leaves
lilac
lettuce
lamb
lawn mower
lily
leprechaun

### Medial
tulip
violet
dandelion
daylight
fertilizer
Queen Anne's Lace
pollen
umbrella
violet
tiller

### Final
April
baby animal
daffodil
cardinal
drizzle

soil
shovel
ball
tadpole
bluebell
eggshell
petal
puddle
baseball

### Blends
plant
sunflower
flower
clover
flowerpot
spring cleaning
bluebird
butterfly
blossom
fly
April Fool's Day
marigold
seedling
pot of gold

## /k/ and /k/ blends

### Initial
cardinal
Queen Anne's Lace
carrot
carnation
cow
calf
kite

### Medial
picnic
orchid
chicken
jacket
buttercup

### Final
picnic
spring break
lilac
chick

### Blends
clover

#BK-272  Year-Round Literature  •  ©1999 Super Duper® Publications  •  1-800-277-8737  •  www.superduperinc.com

# Spring Articulation & Vocabulary Word Lists (Cont.)

## /k/ and /k/ blends cont.

Queen Anne's Lace
spring cleaning
ski
ski pole
Christmas
Christmas Tree
Santa Claus
Ice skating
Easter Basket

## /g/ and /g/ blends

### Initial
garden

### Medial
marigold
eggshells
snapdragon
pot of gold

### Final
pig
egg
frog

### Blends
grow
green grass
Piglet
Easter eggs

## /th/

### Initial
thermos
third base

### Medial
weather
feather
spring clothing
Mother's Day

### Final
hyacinth

## /sh/

### Initial
short
shirt

shovel
sheep
shoes
shorts
short stop

### Medial
fishing
eggshells
carnation

### Final
fish
squash
radish

## /ch/

### Initial
chickens
chick
cherry tree
chirp

### Medial
orchard
kitchen
catcher
artichoke

### Final
March
hatch
branch

## /m/ and /m/ blends

### Initial
March
Mother's Day
marigold

### Medial
tomato
animal
hummingbird
lawn mower
home run

### Final
warm
worm
broom
blossom
lamb

## Blends
umbrella

## /p/ and /p/ blends

### Initial
pig
piglet
puppy
pollen
picnic
pants
petals
puddle
pansy
pot of gold

### Medial
tadpoles
snapdragon
flowerpot

### Final
sheep
tulip
buttercup

### Blends
April
April Fool's Day
plow
plant
spring cleaning
spring
sprout
spring break

## /b/ and /b/ blends

### Initial
baby animals
bat
ball
bee
bird
buttercup
butterfly
bunny
basket

### Medial
rainbow
rain boots
baseball field
green beans
robin
hummingbird

Easter basket
Easter bunny
strawberry

### Blends
blossom
bluebell
branch
breeze
spring break
umbrella

## /f/ and /f/ blends

### Initial
feather
food
fur
foal
fertilizer
four leaf clover

### Medial
daffodils
April Fool's Day

### Final
calf
leaf

### Blends
flower
flowerpot
frogs
fly
sunflower
wildflowers

## /v/ and /v/ blends

### Initial
violet

### Medial
clover
spring fever

### Blends
candles
short sleeves
leaves
shovel

# Vocabulary Pictures

**Instructions:** _____

_____

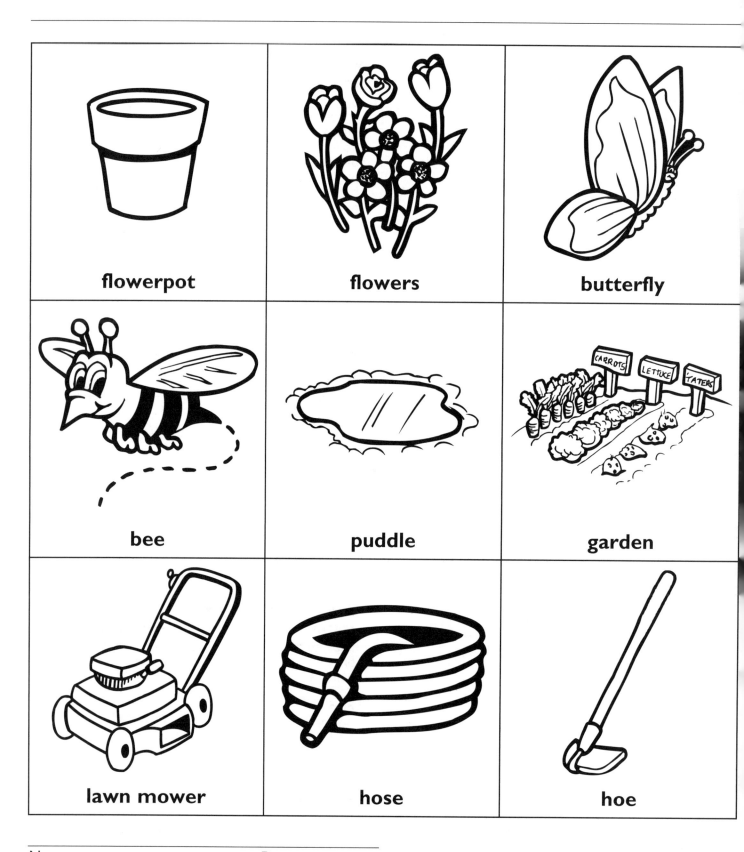

| | | |
|---|---|---|
| flowerpot | flowers | butterfly |
| bee | puddle | garden |
| lawn mower | hose | hoe |

Name _____      Date _____

# Vocabulary Pictures

**Instructions:** _____

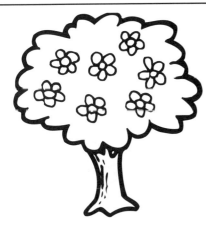
tree with buds

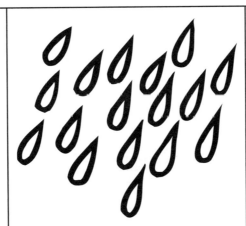
rain

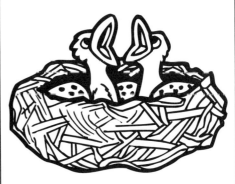
baby birds in nest

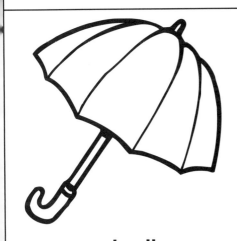
umbrella

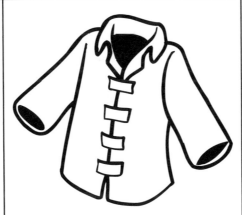
raincoat

rainbow

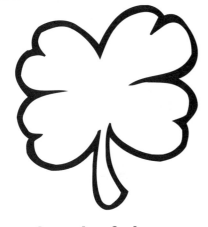
four leaf clover

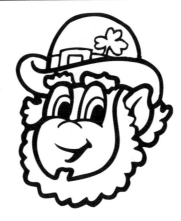
leprechaun

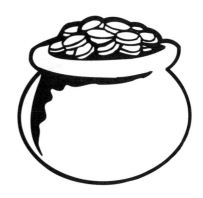
pot of gold

Name _____    Date _____

Speech-Language Pathologist      Helper's Signature

# Vocabulary Pictures

**Instructions:** _____

_____

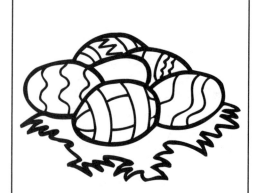

**Easter eggs**

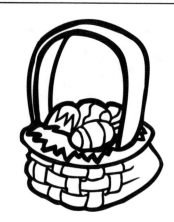

**Easter basket**

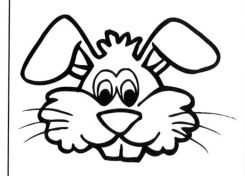

**Easter bunny**

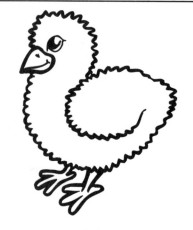

**chick**

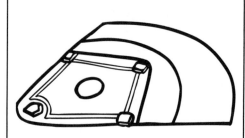

**baseball field**

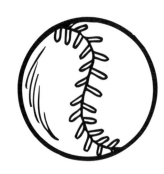

**baseball**

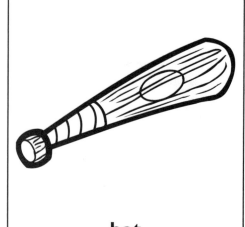

**bat**

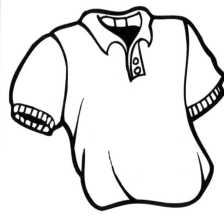

**short sleeve shirt**

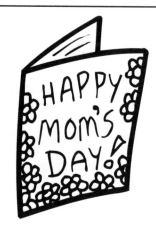

**Mother's Day card**

Name _____

Date _____

Speech-Language Pathologist

Helper's Signature

#BK-272 Year-Round Literature • ©1999 Super Duper® Publications • 1-800-277-8737 • www.superduperinc.com

# Story Pattern

**Name:** _____

_____

_____

_____

_____

_____

_____

_____

_____

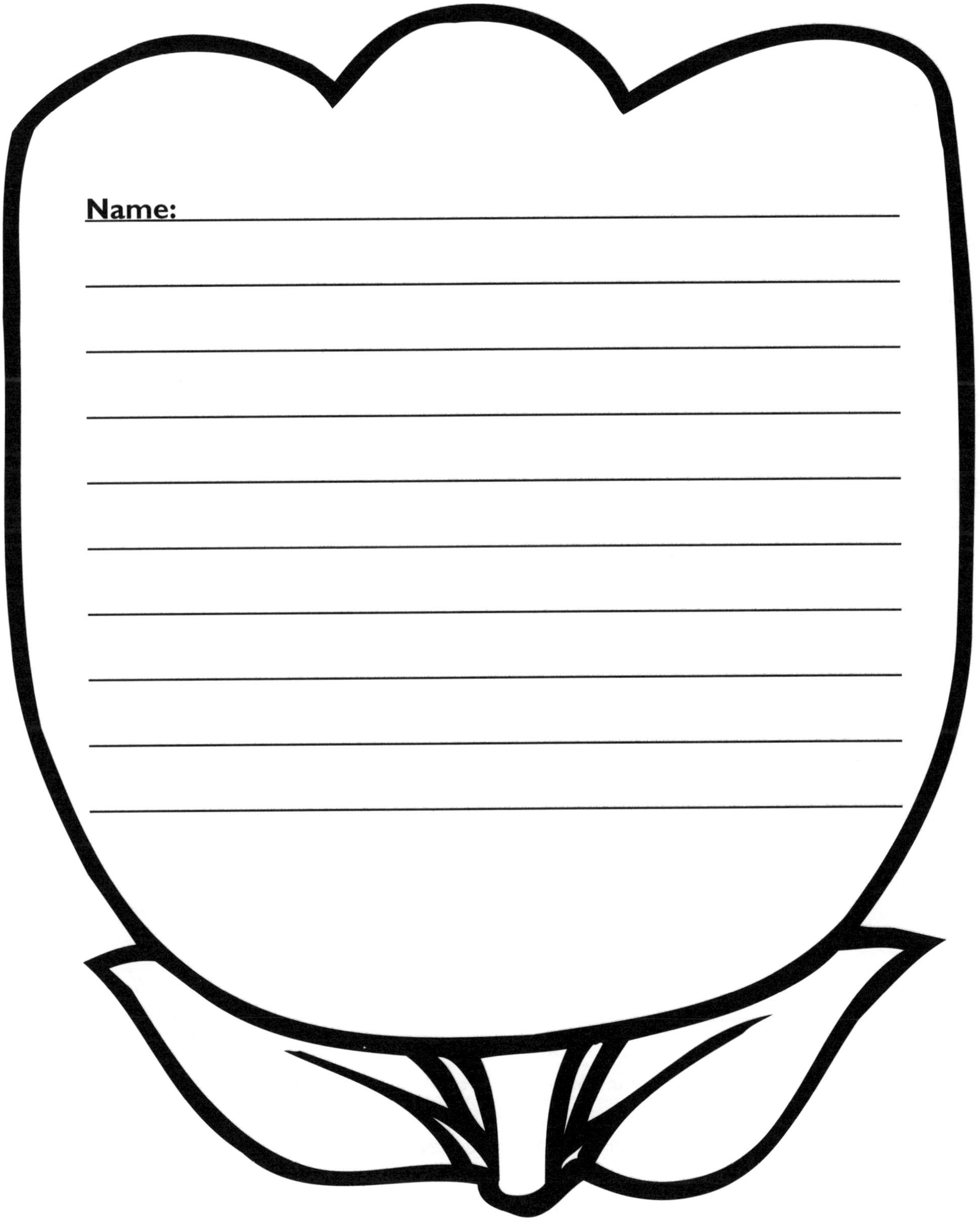

Name                                Date

Speech-Language Pathologist                        Helper's Signature

# The Spring Snowman

adapted by Jill Barnes, story and illustrations by Fusako Ishinabe

This is a wonderful story about a snowman who goes through the seasonal change from winter to spring. Once the snowman melts, a snowman made of beautiful, white flowers appears.

**Language Expansion:** The following questions can be used to address students' recall of this book or to expand upon concepts addressed in this book.

## Definition
1. What is a snowman?
2. What is a mountain?
3. What is spring?
4. What is a flower?
5. What does melting mean?

## Function
1. What is a snowman used for?
2. What are flowers used for?
3. What is snow used for?
4. What is the sun for?
5. What are mountains for?

## Category
1. Name three animals that visited the snowman.
2. Name three things you can see in the forest.
3. Name three things that make blossoms.
4. Name three games you can play in the spring.
5. Name three things you can use to decorate a snowman.

## Description
1. Tell me three things about flowers.
2. Tell me three things about trees.
3. Tell me three things about the snowman.
4. Tell me about three games you can play in the spring.
5. Tell me three things about a mountain.

## Vocabulary
Make a sentence using the following words.
1. mountain
2. snow
3. blossom
4. spring
5. forest

## Rhyming
Name a rhyming word for each word below.
1. snow
2. spring
3. tree
4. white
5. fun

## Sequencing
As your students sequence the events in this story, use this list as a guide.
1. A snowman stands all alone on a mountain.
2. Animals on their way down the mountain stop and wave at the snowman.
3. The animals tell the snowman that spring is coming.
4. The snowman melts as the weather gets warm.
5. The animals go back to see the snowman and find white flowers that bloomed in the sunshine.

#BK-272 Year-Round Literature • ©1999 Super Duper® Publications • 1-800-277-8737 • www.superduperinc.com

# Hopper Hunts for Spring
## by Marcus Pfister

Hopper, the rabbit, hears that spring is coming and thinks that he will have a new playmate. He sets on a journey to find spring and meets several other creatures that are waiting for spring, too. This is a good book to use to teach the concept of hibernation.

**Language Expansion:** The following questions can be used to address students' recall of this book or to expand upon concepts addressed in this book.

## Definition
1. What is spring?
2. What is winter?
3. What is honey?
4. What is a rabbit?
5. What is a bear?

## Function
1. What is a cave used for?
2. What is a hole used for?
3. What is honey used for?
4. What are our eyes for?
5. What are friends for?

## Category
1. Name three animals that Hopper met.
2. Name three foods we eat in the spring.
3. Name the four seasons.
4. Name three things you can do when it gets warmer.
5. Name three plants we see in the spring.

## Description
1. Tell me three things about snow.
2. Tell me three things about the spring.
3. Tell me three things about the bear and its cave.
4. Tell me three things about a rabbit.
5. Tell me three things about honey.

## Vocabulary
Make a sentence using the following words.
1. hole
2. cave
3. honey
4. bear
5. friend

## Rhyming
Name a rhyming word for each word below.
1. honey
2. cave
3. hole
4. eye
5. bear

## Sequencing
As your students sequence the events in this story, use this list as a guide.
1. Hopper's mother tells him that spring is coming and he thinks that spring is an animal.
2. Hopper goes to look for spring.
3. Hopper looks for spring in a hole, a cave, and a tree.
4. Hopper cannot find spring.
5. Hopper's mother tells him that spring is not an animal but a time of year.

# The Very Hungry Caterpillar
## by Eric Carle

This is a story about a caterpillar that eats and eats until he has a stomachache.  Then, the caterpillar forms a cocoon and stays there for several days.  In the end, the caterpillar turns into a beautiful butterfly.

**Language Expansion:**  The following questions can be used to address students' recall of this book or to expand upon concepts addressed in this book.

## Definition
1. What is an egg?
2. What is a caterpillar?
3. What is a stomachache?
4. What is a cocoon?
5. What is a butterfly?

## Function
1. What is a cocoon used for?
2. What are oranges used for?
3. What is cheese used for?
4. What is the sun used for?
5. What is the moon used for?

## Category
1. Name three kinds of fruit.
2. Name three different foods that the caterpillar ate.
3. Name three days of the week.
4. Name three things that you can see in the sky.
5. Name three desserts you like to eat.

## Description
1. Tell me three things about a caterpillar.
2. Tell me three things about a butterfly.
3. Tell me three things about a leaf.
4. Tell me three things about a cocoon.
5. Tell me three things about the sun.

## Vocabulary
Make a sentence using the following words.
1. cocoon
2. butterfly
3. caterpillar
4. strawberry
5. ice cream cone

## Rhyming
Name a rhyming word for each word below.
1. egg
2. cheese
3. moon
4. fruit
5. berry

## Sequencing
As your students sequence the events in this story, use this list as a guide.
1. A caterpillar hatches from an egg.
2. The caterpillar is very hungry and goes to look for some food.
3. The caterpillar eats lots of food and gets very big.
4. The caterpillar makes a cocoon and stays inside for more than two weeks.
5. The cocoon opens and out comes a beautiful butterfly.

 #BK-272  Year-Round Literature  •  ©1999 Super Duper® Publications  •  1-800-277-8737  •  www.superduperinc.com

# Spring Articulation and Language Games

(The following games can be used with the articulation and vocabulary word list or the literature language questions.)

## Flower Matching Game

Photocopy two copies of the flower pattern (page 52). Color the flowers, cut them apart, and laminate them. Lay the cards facedown and allow each student to turn over two cards. If the cards don't match, the student must choose one of the cards to name and describe using good speech and language and then put both cards facedown. If the cards match, the student must tell about the flower by naming it and then describing it using good speech and language. Then, the student may keep the matching pair. Continue taking turns until all of the flowers have been matched. The student with the most matches is the winner.

### Team Approach

In order to win the game, the team must be able to match all of the flowers by the end of the therapy session. Put all the matches in the team flowerpot.

## Parts of a Flower Game

Photocopy, color, and laminate the flower game board (page 53). Then, photocopy the student sheet (page 54) for each student. (You can photocopy front and back to save paper and use the back side with the next therapy group.) Make a game die using a penny. Put a piece of masking tape on both sides and write a "2" on one side and a "3" on the other side with permanent ink.

Discuss the different parts of a flower shown on the game board. The goal is for each student to get each part to complete the flower on the student sheet. Then, give each child a student sheet and a pencil. After the student makes a sentence with a spring word containing his/her sound or answers a spring language question, the student may flip the penny die, move the allotted spaces, and then draw the flower part of the student sheet.

### Language Extension

After completing the flower, ask the student to name the parts and tell the purpose of each part.

## Kite Game

Photocopy, color, cut out, and laminate the kite pattern (page 55). Turn the cards facedown. After a student makes a sentence with a spring word containing his/her sound or answers a spring language question, the student chooses one kite card. If the kite has directions, the student must follow the directions. If the kite is blank, the student may keep the kite. The student with the most kites at the end of the game is the winner.

### Team Approach

In order to win the game, the team must earn a designated number of kites. For example, the team must have 15 kites by the end of the class to win.

## Chick Hatching from an Egg Game

Photocopy chick hatching pattern (page 56) on yellow or white construction paper. Color and cut out chick hatchings. Write the number "1," "2," or "3" on the back of 16 eggs. Write the number 10 on four eggs. Laminate the eggs. After a student makes a sentence with a spring word containing his/her sound or answers a spring language question, the student may draw an egg. The number on the back is the number of points the student received on the score sheet for the turn. The student with the most points wins.

### Team Approach

In order to win the game, the team must earn a designated number of points. For example, to win the team must have 30 points by the end of the class.

## Blooming Game

Make one copy of the flower pattern (page 57) for each student. Color, laminate, and cut out all the flowers. Cut a long piece of green bulletin board paper (about 6 feet long) for each student so that it resembles a flower stem. Lay the stems on the floor and tell the students to stand at the end of a stem holding their large flowers. (Or you can attach a string to the flower so that it hangs like a necklace around each student's neck.) The small flowers are direction cards. After a student makes a sentence with a spring word containing his/her sound or answers a spring language question, the student may choose a direction card. The direction card will tell the student to move forward a certain number of steps, backward a certain number of steps, or to remain in place. The student who gets to the end of the stem first may put his/her flower atop the stem and is the winner of the game.

### Language Extension

After completing the game, ask the students to brainstorm as many types of flowers as they can. Write the flower names on a piece of paper and encourage the students to find pictures of these flowers.

# Flower Matching Game

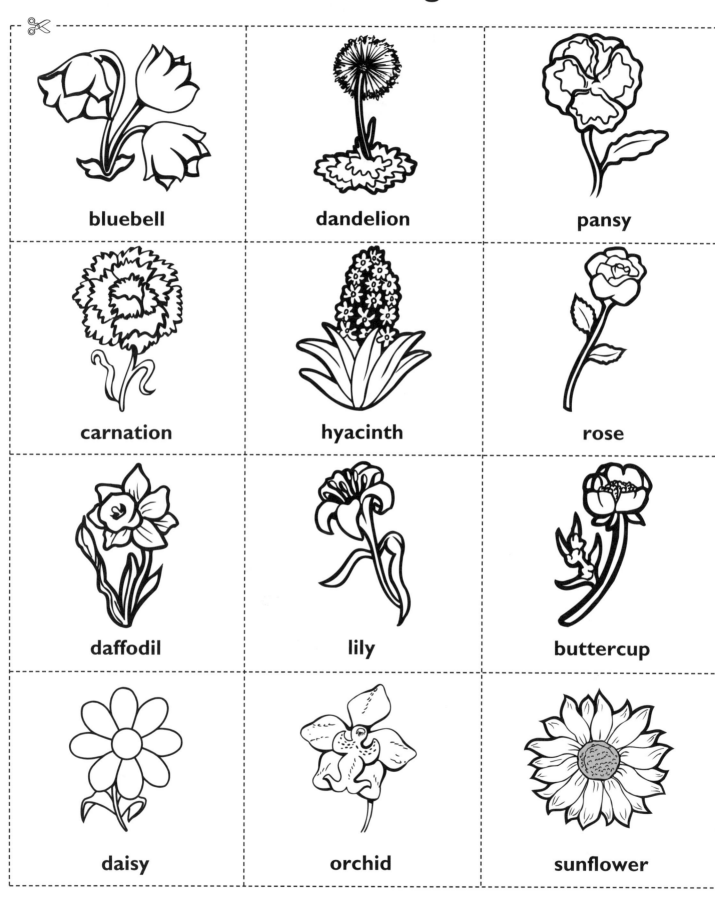

bluebell

dandelion

pansy

carnation

hyacinth

rose

daffodil

lily

buttercup

daisy

orchid

sunflower

#BK-272  Year-Round Literature  •  ©1999 Super Duper® Publications  •  1-800-277-8737  •  www.superduperinc.com

# Parts of a Flower Game Board

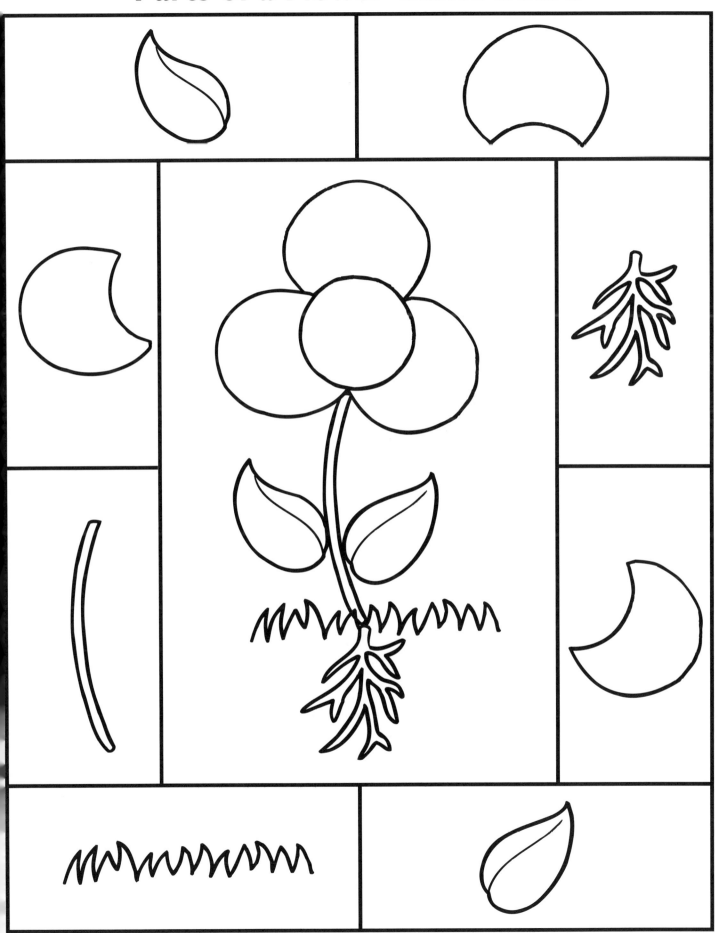

# Parts of a Flower Student Sheet

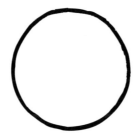

#BK-272  Year-Round Literature  •  ©1999 Super Duper® Publications  •  1-800-277-8737  •  www.superduperinc.com

# Kites Game

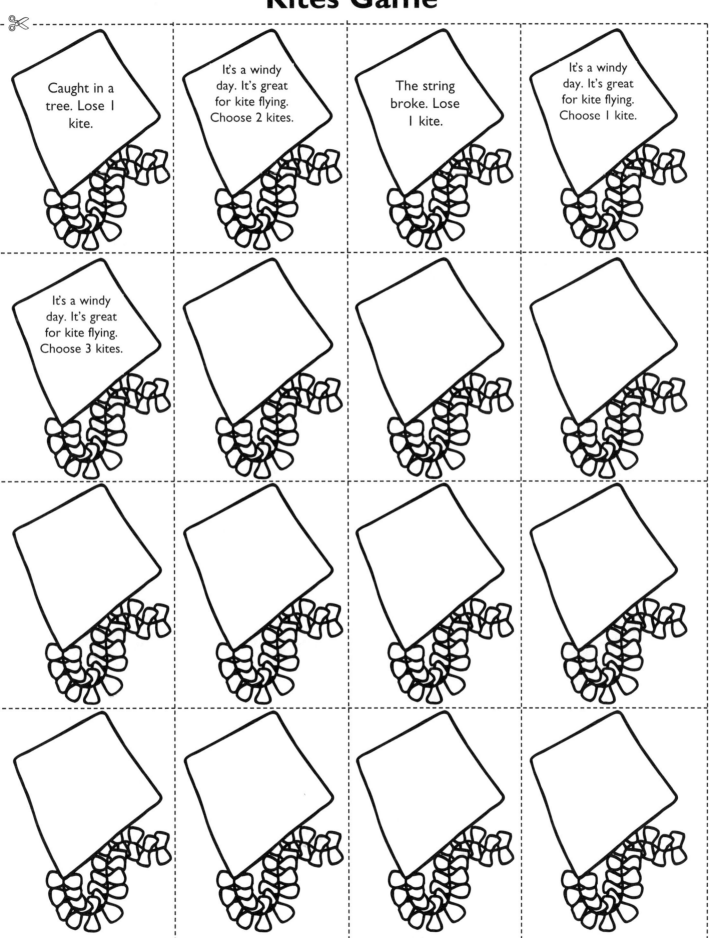

Caught in a tree. Lose 1 kite.

It's a windy day. It's great for kite flying. Choose 2 kites.

The string broke. Lose 1 kite.

It's a windy day. It's great for kite flying. Choose 1 kite.

It's a windy day. It's great for kite flying. Choose 3 kites.

# Chick Hatching From an Egg Game

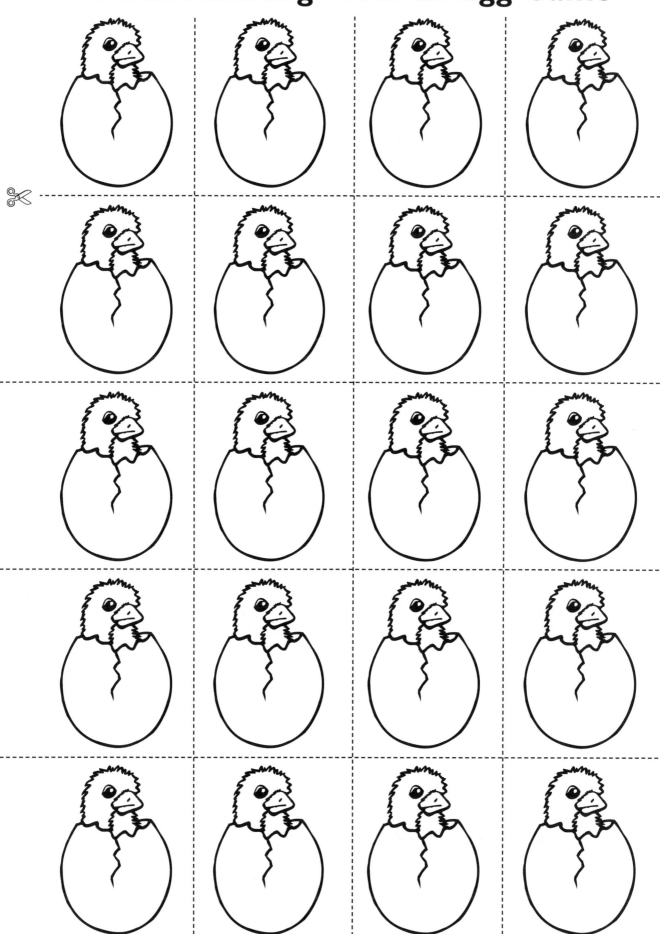

#BK-272  Year-Round Literature  •  ©1999 Super Duper® Publications  •  1-800-277-8737  •  www.superduperinc.com

# Blooming Game

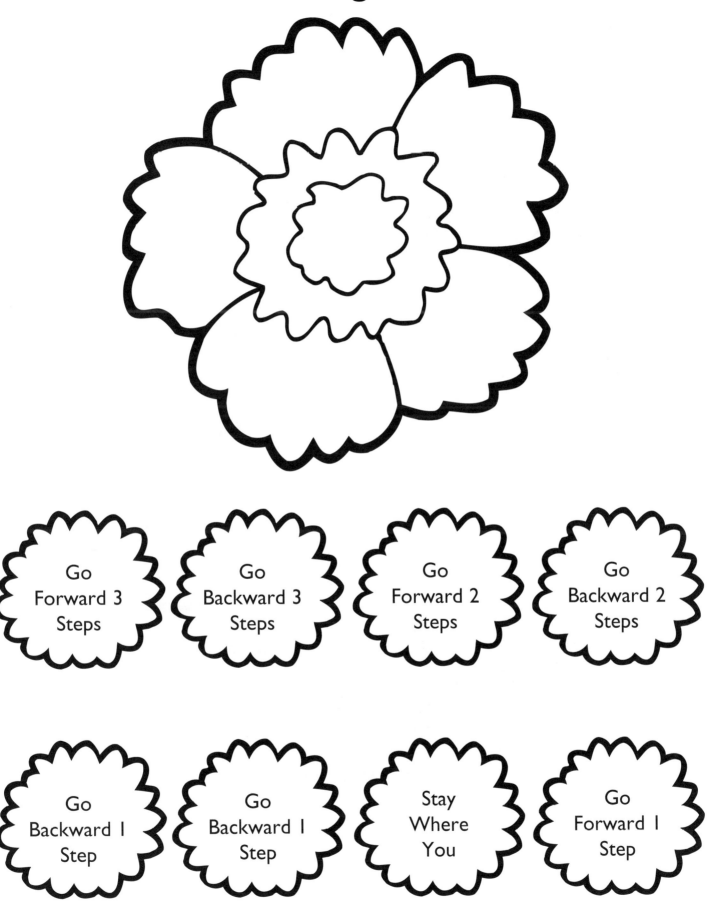

# Blooming Good Speech

Write words with the _____ sound on each flower petal.  Then, make a sentence with each word out loud using your good speech.

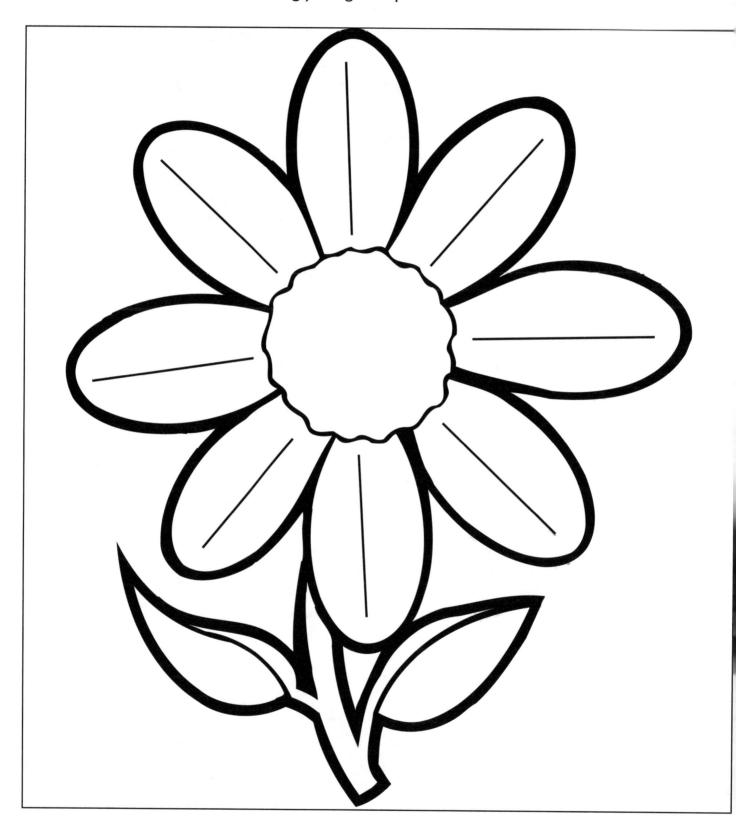

Name _____        Date _____

_____
Speech-Language Pathologist

_____
Helper's Signature

#BK-272  Year-Round Literature  •  ©1999 Super Duper® Publications  •  1-800-277-8737  •  www.superduperinc.com

# Kite Flying

In the spring when the weather is windy, it's fun to fly a kite. Put the pictures below in the correct order for making a kite to fly. Then, tell about each picture using your good speech.

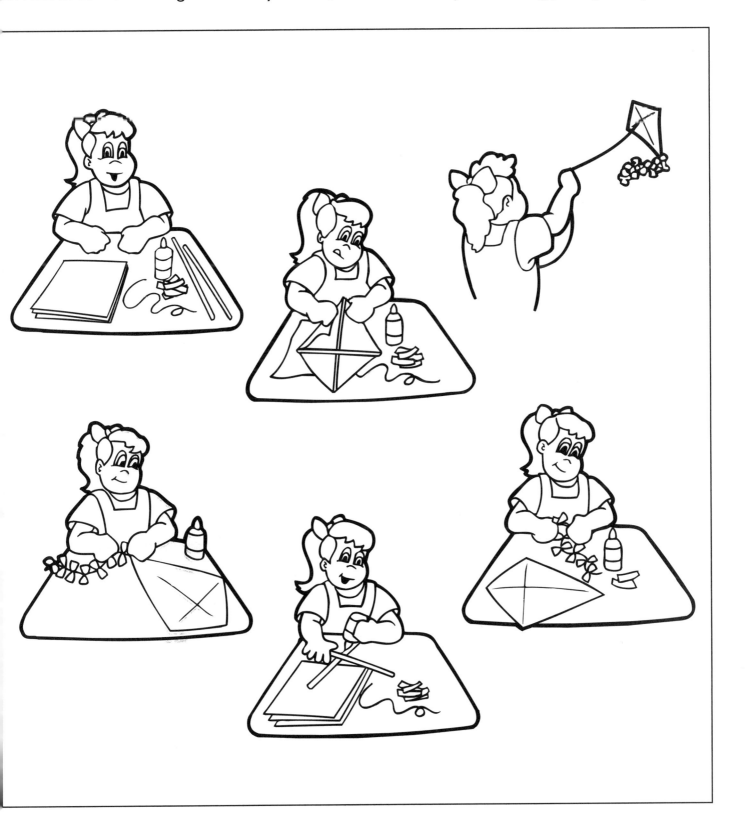

Name _____ Date _____

Speech-Language Pathologist

Helper's Signature

# It's Spring!

Look at the pictures below.  Which pictures go together?  Draw a line from one picture to the picture it goes with.  Then, tell why the pictures go together using your good speech.

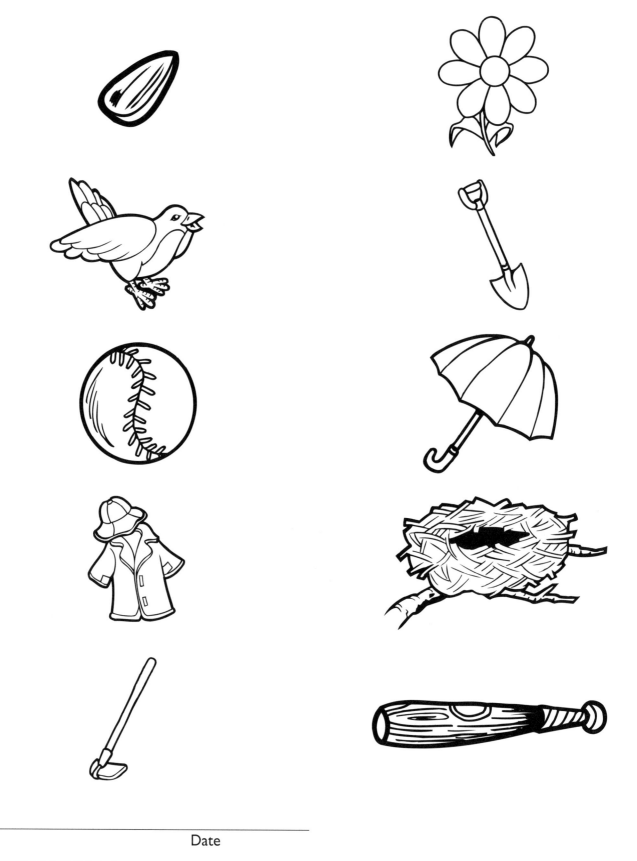

# Summer

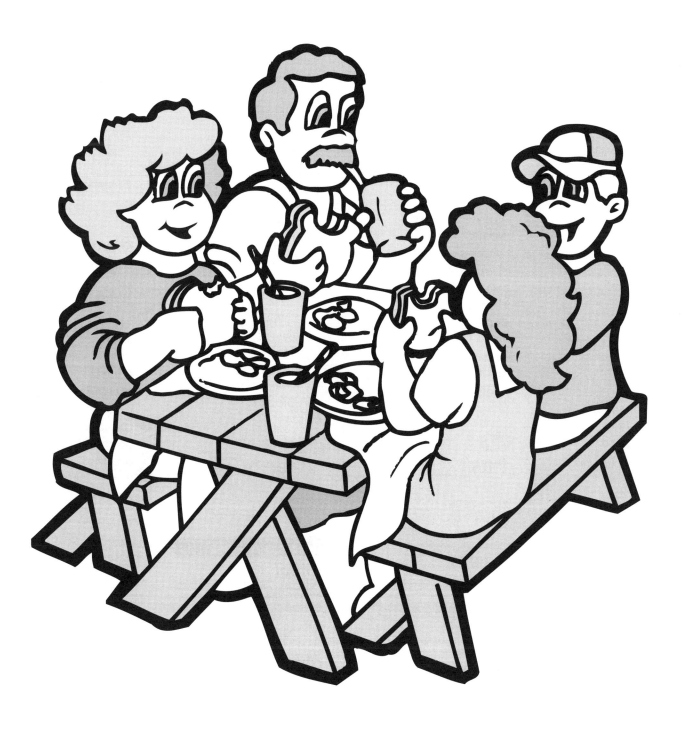

# Summer Articulation & Vocabulary Word Lists

These word lists are a good resource for articulation and/or vocabulary building activities.

## /r/ and /r/ blends

### Initial
rain
rainbow

### Medial
butterflies
starfish
motorboat
water-skiing
watermelon
fireworks

### Final
summer
hot weather
thunder
caterpillar
sunflower
September
car
lawn chair

### Blends
ice cream
sunscreen
grill
strawberry
grape
crab
Fourth of July
shorts
short-sleeved shirt
sunburn
thunderstorm
lifeguard
diving board

## /s/ and /s/ blends

### Initial
summer
sun
sandals
sand
September
sun hat
sunburn
sea gulls
sunflower
seashell

### Medial
ice cream cone
popsicle
sunflower seeds
sunglasses
bicycle

### Final
flip-flops
shorts
grapes

### Blends
swimming pool
swimming
swimming suit
splash
starfish
sleeveless shirt
strawberry
water-skiing
short-sleeved shirt
sunscreen
thunderstorm
August
outside
seashell
sandcastle
fireworks

## /z/

### Initial
zoo
zookeeper
zebra

### Final
butterflies
bees
long days
shells
sea gulls
sunflower seeds
seeds

## /l/ and /l/ blends

### Initial
long days
lifeguard
lightning
lawn chair

### Medial
caterpillar
sailboat
watermelon
July
Fourth of July

### Final
beach ball
pool
grill
sea gull
sandcastle
seashell

### Blends
butterfly
sunglasses
flip flops
short-sleeved shirt
sleeveless shirt
sun block
clam
splash
shells
sandals
popsicle
bicycle

## /k/ and /k/ blends

### Initial
camping
canoe
car

### Medial
picnic
vacation
sandcastle

## Blends
crab
clam
ice cream
sunscreen
water skiing
fireworks
popsicle
bicycle

## /g/ and /g/ blends

### Medial
lifeguard
sea gull
August

### Final
flag

### Blends
sunglasses
grill
grapes

## /th/

### Initial
thermometer
thunder
thunderstorm
theme park
thermos

### Medial
warm weather
summer clothing
bathing suit
Fourth of July
Father's Day

#BK-272 Year-Round Literature • ©1999 Super Duper® Publications • 1-800-277-8737 • www.superduperinc.com

# Summer Articulation & Vocabulary Word Lists (Cont.)

## /sh/

### Initial
shells
shorts
short-sleeved
shirt

### Medial
vacation
fishing pole
suntan lotion
splashing
seashell

### Final
starfish
fish

## /ch/

### Initial
chocolate ice cream
chores
chocolate cake
cherry pie
chocolate
chip

### Medial
beach ball
lawn chair
chocolate chip cookies

### Final
beach

## /m/ and /m/ blends

### Initial
motorboat

### Medial
swimming pool
swimming suit
watermelon
humid

### Final
swim
ice cream
thunderstorm
clam

### Blends
September
camping
warm

## /p/ and /p/ blends

### Initial
picnic
pool

### Medial
popsicle
flip-flops
camping
caterpillar

### Blends
splashing
September
grapes

## /b/ and /b/ blends

### Initial
bee
butterfly
beach
beach ball
bicycle

### Medial
beach ball
sailboat
motorboat
skateboard
sunburn
strawberry

### Final
crab

### Blends
sun block

## /f/ and /f/ blends

### Initial
fish
fishing
fishing pole
Fourth of July
fireworks
Father's Day
family

### Medial
starfish

### Blends
flip-flops
butterfly
flag

## /v/ and /v/ blends

### Initial
vacation

### Medial
diving board

### Blends
waves

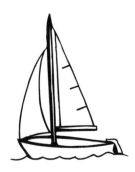

# Vocabulary Pictures

**Instructions:** _____

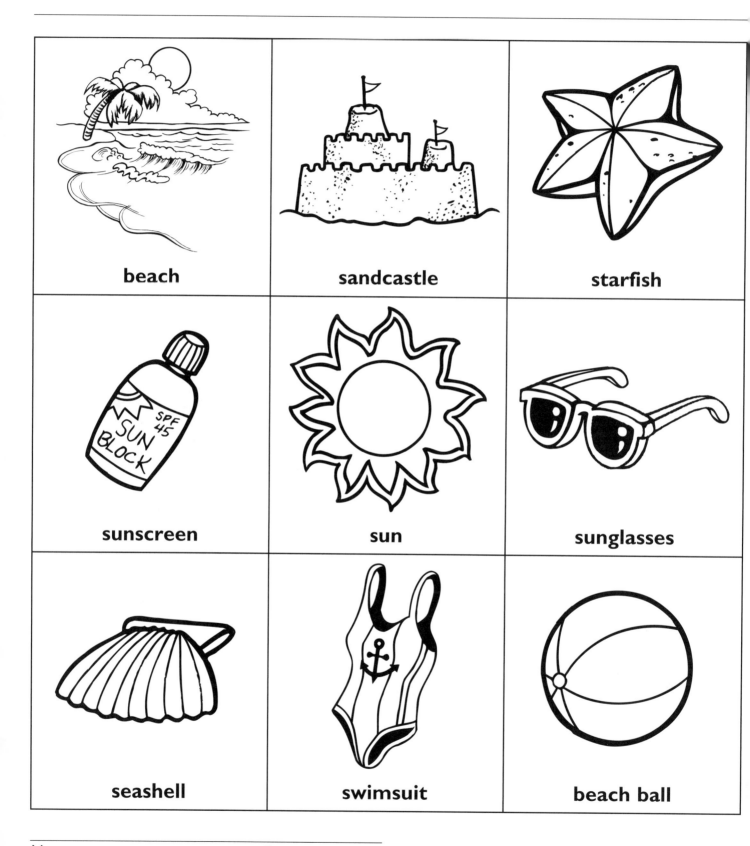

| | | |
|---|---|---|
| **beach** | **sandcastle** | **starfish** |
| **sunscreen** | **sun** | **sunglasses** |
| **seashell** | **swimsuit** | **beach ball** |

Name _____ Date _____

Speech-Language Pathologist                    Helper's Signature

#BK-272  Year-Round Literature  •  ©1999 Super Duper® Publications  •  1-800-277-8737  •  www.superduperinc.com

# Vocabulary Pictures

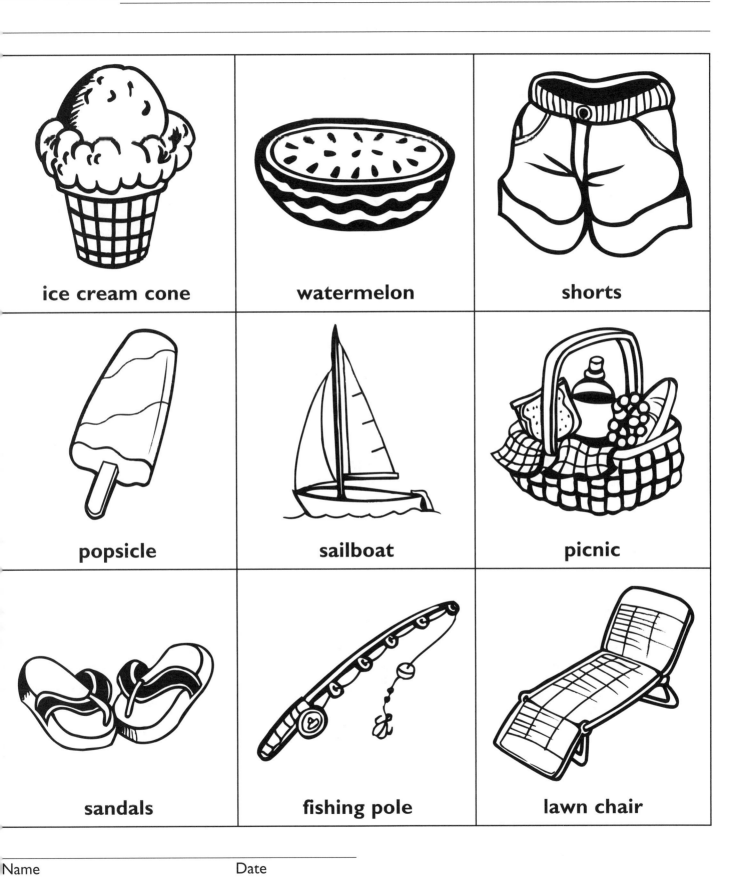

| | | |
|---|---|---|
| ice cream cone | watermelon | shorts |
| popsicle | sailboat | picnic |
| sandals | fishing pole | lawn chair |

Name _____     Date _____

Speech-Language Pathologist          Helper's Signature

# Vocabulary Pictures

**Instructions:** _____

_____

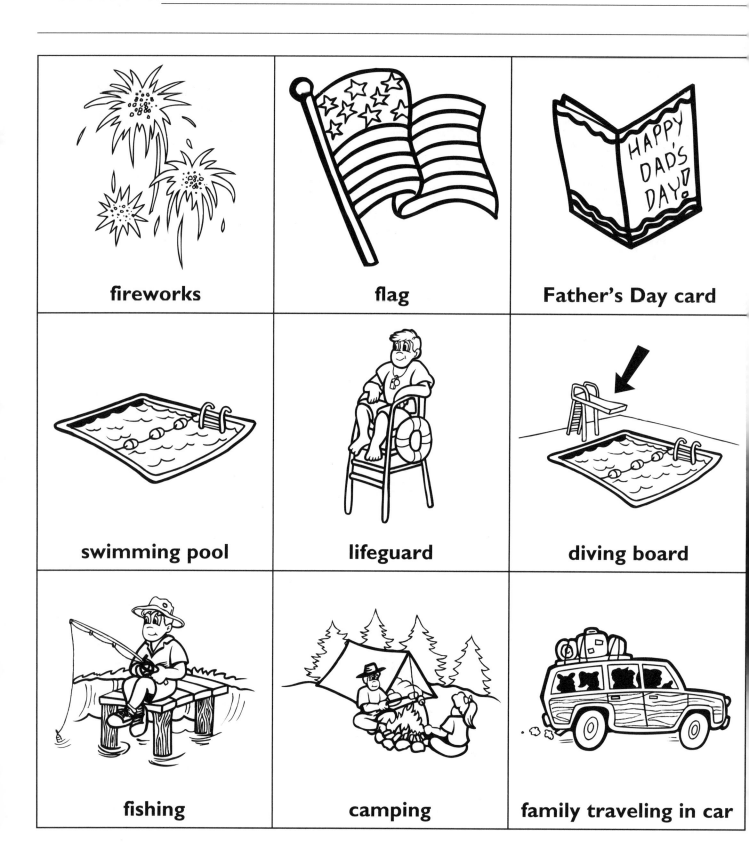

fireworks

flag

Father's Day card

swimming pool

lifeguard

diving board

fishing

camping

family traveling in car

Name _____  Date _____

Speech-Language Pathologist

Helper's Signature

#BK-272  Year-Round Literature  •  ©1999 Super Duper® Publications  •  1-800-277-8737  •  www.superduperinc.com

# Story Pattern

Instructions: _____

**Name:** _____

_____

_____

_____

_____

_____

_____

_____

_____

_____

Name                              Date

Speech-Language Pathologist                    Helper's Signature

# Sunflower House
## by Eve Bunting

This is a story about a family who plants a circle of sunflowers so that when they are grown, it's a sunflower house. When summer is over, the sunflowers wilt. Then the children realize they can gather the seeds so they can have sunflowers next summer.

**Language Expansion:** The following questions can be used to address students' recall of this book or to expand upon concepts addressed in this book.

## Definition
1. What are weeds?
2. What is a sunflower?
3. What is a stem?
4. What is a petal?
5. What is summer?

## Function
1. What is a seed used for?
2. How are the strings and stick used?
3. What is a stem used for?
4. How did they use the sunflower?
5. What are sunflower seeds used for?

## Category
1. Name three kinds of flowers.
2. Name three parts of a sunflower.
3. Name three things the children did in the sunflower house.
4. Name three kinds of birds.
5. Name the four seasons.

## Description
1. Tell me three things about the summer.
2. Tell me three things about a seed.
3. Tell me three things about a sunflower.
4. Tell me three things about the sunflower house.
5. Tell me three things about warm weather.

## Vocabulary
Make a sentence using the following words.
1. weeds
2. mammoth flower
3. stem
4. petal
5. summer

## Rhyming
Name a rhyming word for each word below.
1. string
2. seed
3. grow
4. child
5. flowers

## Sequencing
As your students sequence the events in this story, use this list as a guide.
1. The little boy plants his sunflower seeds in a circle.
2. The little boy waters the seeds and the sunflowers grow in a circle.
3. The circle of sunflowers makes a sunflower house for the kids to play in.
4. When fall arrives, the sunflowers begin to wilt.
5. The children collect the seeds so they can have sunflowers next summer.

#BK-272  Year-Round Literature • ©1999 Super Duper® Publications • 1-800-277-8737 • www.superduperinc.com

# How I Spent My Summer Vacation
## by Marc Teague

Wallace Bleff's teacher has the students in the class tell about their summer vacations. Wallace tells of his exciting adventures out west. He boarded the train to visit Aunt Fern, but was captured by cowboys. The book continues with the happenings of Wallace's exciting vacation.

**Language Expansion:** The following questions can be used to address students' recall of this book or to expand upon concepts addressed in this book.

## Definition

1. What is summer?
2. What is a vacation?
3. What is your imagination?
4. What is a cowboy?
5. What is a stampede?

## Function

1. What is a vacation for?
2. What is a train used for?
3. What is a rope used for?
4. What is a band for?
5. What did Wallace Bleff use the tablecloth for?

## Category

1. Name three things to do in the summer.
2. Name three things to travel in.
3. Name three places to go on vacation.
4. Name three things a cowboy wears.
5. Name three things a cowboy does.

## Description

1. Tell me three things about the summer.
2. Tell me three things about a vacation.
3. Tell me three things about a train.
4. Tell me three things about a cowboy.
5. Name the four seasons.

## Vocabulary

Make a sentence using the following words.
1. vacation
2. imagination
3. plains
4. cowboy
5. stampede

## Rhyming

Name a rhyming word for each word below.
1. train
2. teacher
3. west
4. rope
5. band

## Sequencing

As your students sequence the events in this story, use this list as a guide.
1. Wallace heads west for summer vacation.
2. Wallace imagines that he is caught by cowboys who take him to cow camp.
3. The cowboys and Wallace go to Aunt Fern's for a barbecue.
4. At the barbecue, the cattle begin charging towards Wallace.
5. Wallace uses the tablecloth like a matador, and the cattle are frightened and stampede away. What a vacation!

# The Relatives Came
## by Cynthia Rylant

This amusing book is about relatives coming to town for summer vacation. It chronicles what goes on during the weeks that the relatives visit. They help tend the garden, fix broken things, and eat up all of the food. Then, the relatives leave and do not return until the following summer.

**Language Expansion:** The following questions can be used to address students' recall of this book or to expand upon concepts addressed in this book.

## Definition
1. What is summer?
2. What are relatives?
3. What is traveling?
4. What is a vacation?
5. What is a garden?

## Function
1. What is a vacation for?
2. What is a car used for?
3. What is an ice chest used for?
4. What is a garden used for?
5. What are instruments used for?

## Category
1. Name three things you can do in the summer.
2. Name three things that you can travel in.
3. Name three of your relatives.
4. Name three things the relatives in the book did.
5. Name the four seasons.

## Description
1. Tell me three things about the summer.
2. Tell me three things about a vacation.
3. Tell me three things about a car.
4. Tell me three things about a garden.
5. Tell me three things about relatives.

## Vocabulary
Make a sentence using the following words.
1. relatives
2. vacation
3. travel
4. garden
5. summer

## Rhyming
Name a rhyming word for each word below.
1. ice
2. car
3. chest
4. came
5. eat

## Sequencing
As your students sequence the events in this story, use this list as a guide.
1. The relatives came to visit family in Virginia for their summer vacation.
2. The relatives laughed, hugged, ate, slept, and had fun.
3. The relatives stayed for weeks and weeks.
4. The relatives loaded up their car.
5. The relatives left and looked forward to coming back the next summer.

#BK-272 Year-Round Literature • ©1999 Super Duper® Publications • 1-800-277-8737 • www.superduperinc.com

# Summer Articulation and Language Games

(The following games can be used with the articulation and vocabulary word list or the literature language questions.)

## Ice Cream Sundae Game

Photocopy the ice cream sundae pattern (page 72). Color the parts, cut them apart, and laminate them. (Hint: Color each scoop of ice cream a different color to represent different ice cream flavors.) Make a sample ice cream sundae so that the students can see what parts they need to make the ice cream sundae. Give each child a bowl piece and put the remaining pieces into a bag. After a student makes a sentence with a summer word containing his/her sound or answers a summer language question, the student may reach into the bag and pull out one sundae piece. (If the child does not have the piece drawn, he/she may keep it for the sundae. If the child does have the piece drawn, he/she must put it back and wait for the next turn.) Whoever completes the ice cream sundae first is the winner.

### Team Approach

In order to win the game, each team member must complete an entire ice cream sundae by the end of class.

## Popsicle Matching Game

Photocopy the popsicle pattern (page 73). Color two popsicles for each color. Glue popsicles to construction paper, cut out, and laminate. Lay all the cards facedown on the table in a pile. After a student makes a sentence with a summer word containing his/her sound or answers a summer language question, the student may choose one popsicle card. The object of the game is to see how many matching colored popsicles each student can collect by the end of class.

### Language Extension

Talk about how popsicles feel and taste. Brainstorm lists of other items that feel cold or taste sweet. Talk about what happens when a popsicle gets warm. What are some other things that melt when they get warm?

## Picnic Game

Make a copy of the picnic pattern (page 74) for each student. Color the pieces, cut them apart, and laminate them. Put a blanket on the floor, give each child a paper plate (or picture of a plate), and tell them that you are going on a pretend picnic. Each student must get a sandwich, an apple, potato chips, a drink, and a cookie from the basket (or bag) to put on the plate by the end of class. After a student makes a sentence with a summer word containing his/her sound or answers a summer language question, the student may reach into the bag and pull out one piece. (If the child does not have the piece drawn, he/she may keep it for his/her plate. If the child does have the piece drawn, he/she must put it back and wait for the next turn.) Whoever completes the picnic plate first is the winner.

### Team Approach

In order to win the game, each team member must fill an entire plate by the end of the class.

## Barrier Game

Color and laminate the barrier game scenes (pages 75 and 76). Copy, color, cut out and laminate the barrier game objects (page 77). Separate the students using a tall box or therapy mirror. Give one team a completed scene. Give the other team the empty scene and objects (page 75). The team with the completed scene must describe to the other team where each object should be placed. The team placing objects is allowed to ask three questions to ensure proper placement. The object is for the team with the empty scene and objects to re-create the completed scene of the other team. The game is ideal for students working on language and listening skills or for those students who are at the sentence or conversation level of articulation therapy.

## Going Camping Game

Make one copy of the trail game board for each student (page 78). Color and laminate each game board. Photocopy on light-colored construction paper, cut out, and laminate the direction cards (page 79). The object of the game is to get the campers to their campsite. After a student makes a sentence with a summer word containing his/her sound or answers a summer language question, the student may choose a direction card. The direction card will tell the student to move forward a certain number of steps on the trail, backwards a certain number of steps on the trail or to remain in place. The student who gets to the campsite first is the winner of the game.

### Language Extension

After completing the game, ask the students to brainstorm the things they might see on a trail through the forest. Then, discuss what you might take on a camping trip and why you might take the items.

# Ice Cream Sundae Game

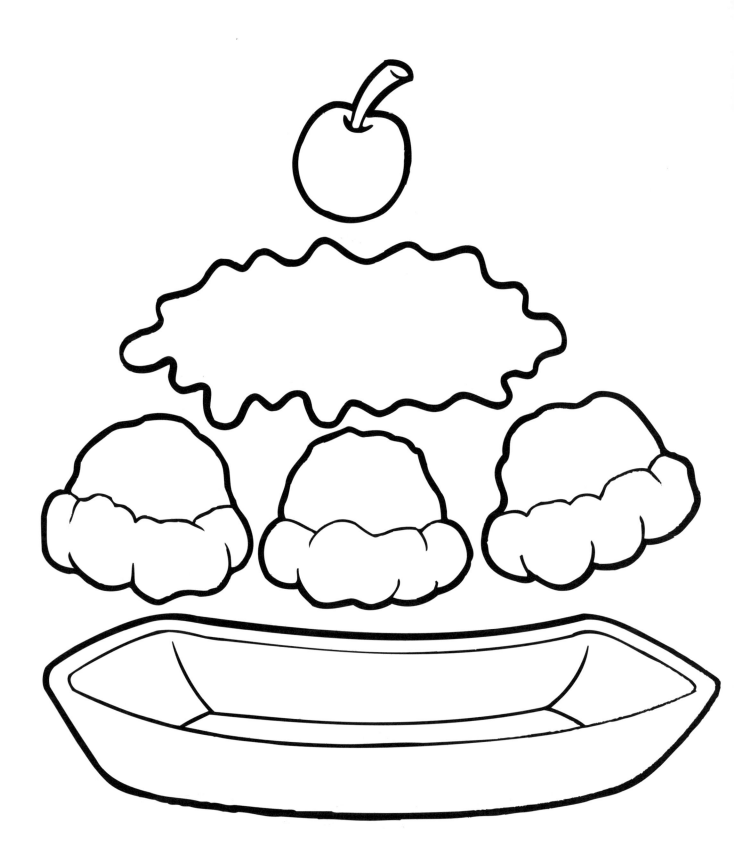

# Popsicle Game

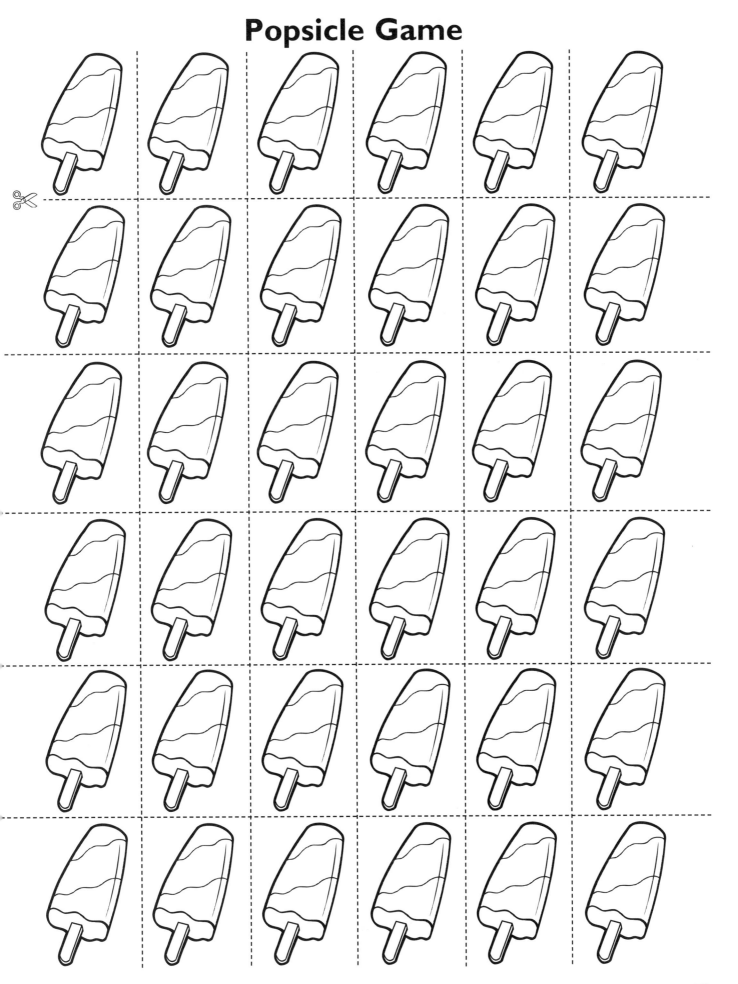

# Picnic Game

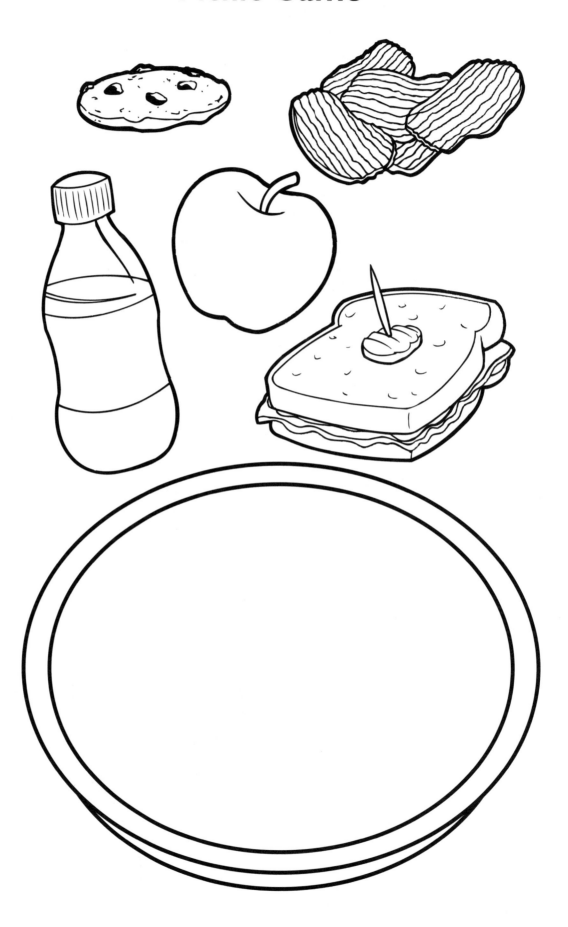

 #BK-272 Year-Round Literature • ©1999 Super Duper® Publications • 1-800-277-8737 • www.superduperinc.com

# Barrier Game

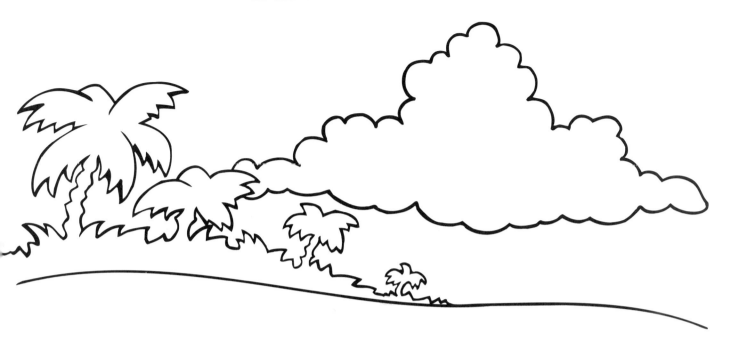

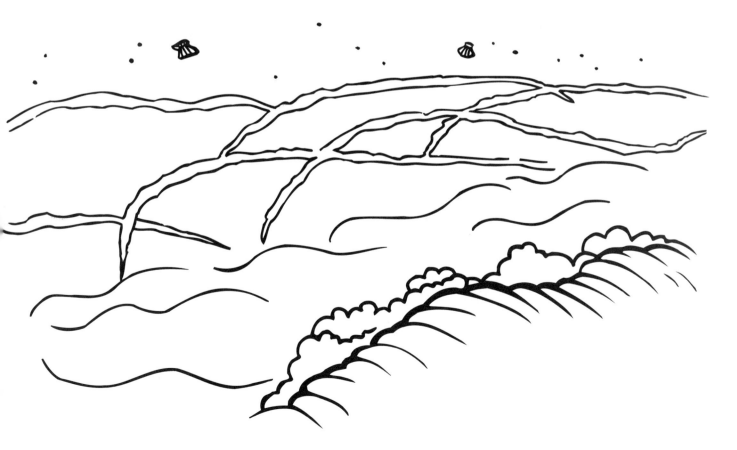

# Barrier Game

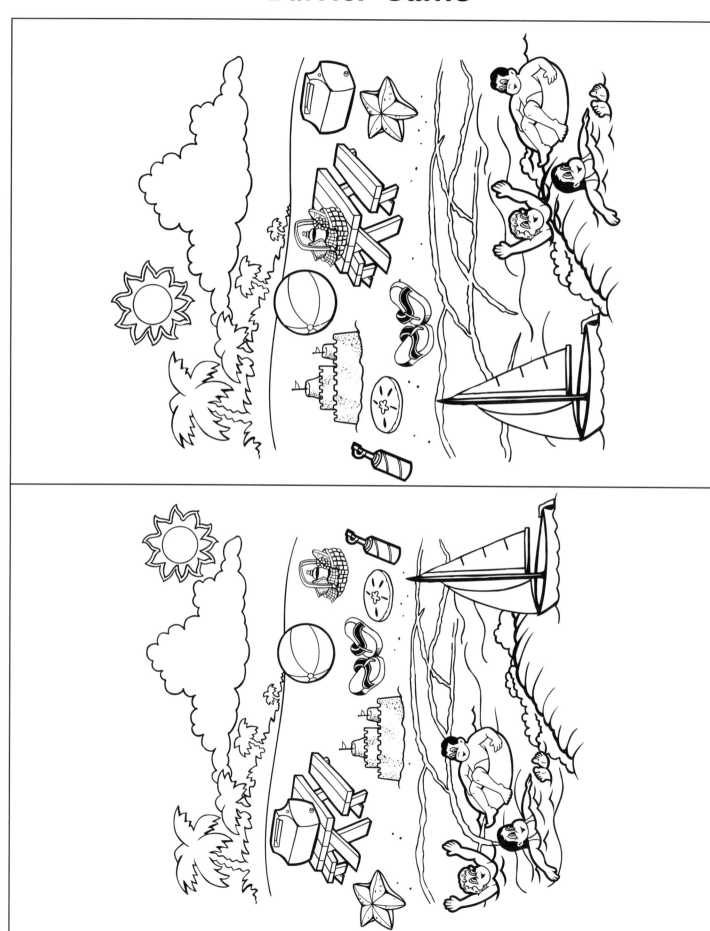

 #BK-272  Year-Round Literature  •  ©1999 Super Duper® Publications  •  1-800-277-8737  •  www.superduperinc.com

# Barrier Game

# Going Camping Game

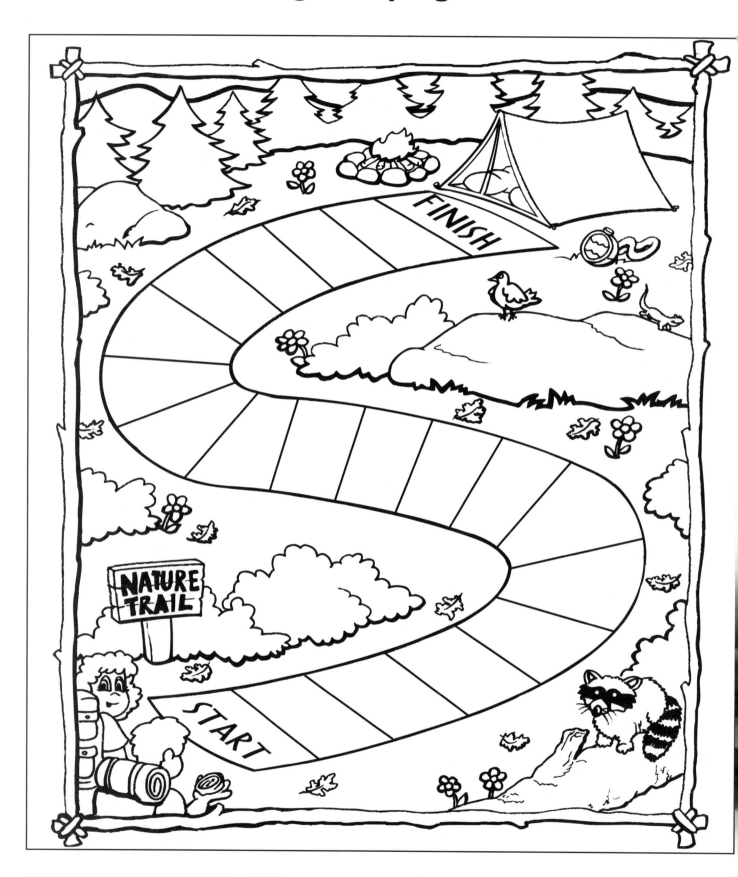

Name _____          Date _____

# Going Camping Game

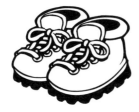

**Wearing good shoes. Go forward 3 steps.**

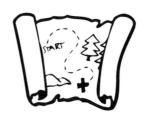

**You read your map. Go forward 1 step.**

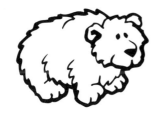

**Ran into a bear. Go backward 3 steps.**

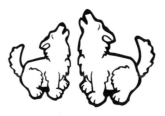

**You hear coyotes howl. Go backward 1 step.**

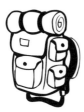

**Packed your backpack well. Go forward 2 steps.**

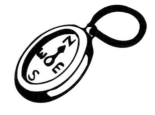

**You can't find your compass. Stay where you are.**

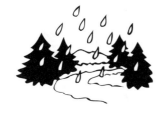

**Trail is slippery from the rain. Go backward 2 steps.**

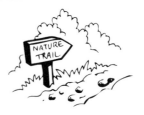

**You are on the right trail. Go forward 1 step.**

# Cool Speech

Write words with the _____ sound in each ice cream cone. Then, make a sentence with each word out loud using your good speech.

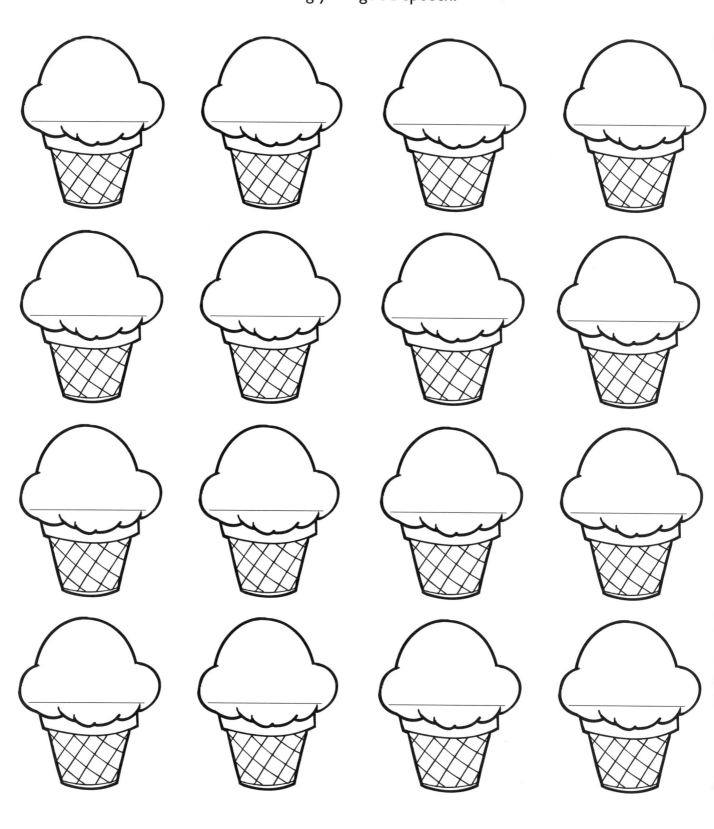

Name _____     Date _____

_____

Speech-Language Pathologist          Helper's Signature

#BK-272  Year-Round Literature  •  ©1999 Super Duper® Publications  •  1-800-277-8737  •  www.superduperinc.com

# Sunny Days

Answer each summer question out loud using your good _____ sound. Keep up the good speech.

Tell about three things that you like to do outside in the summer.

Tell about your favorite summer vacation. Where did you go? What did you do?

Tell about three special foods that you eat in the summer. How do they taste? Why do you like them?

How do you think ice cream is made? What is your favorite kind of ice cream?

Name _____

Date _____

Speech-Language Pathologist _____

Helper's Signature _____

# Summer Fun

Tell what is happening in each summer picture below. Which picture do you think shows the most fun? Why? Tell three things that you like about summer.

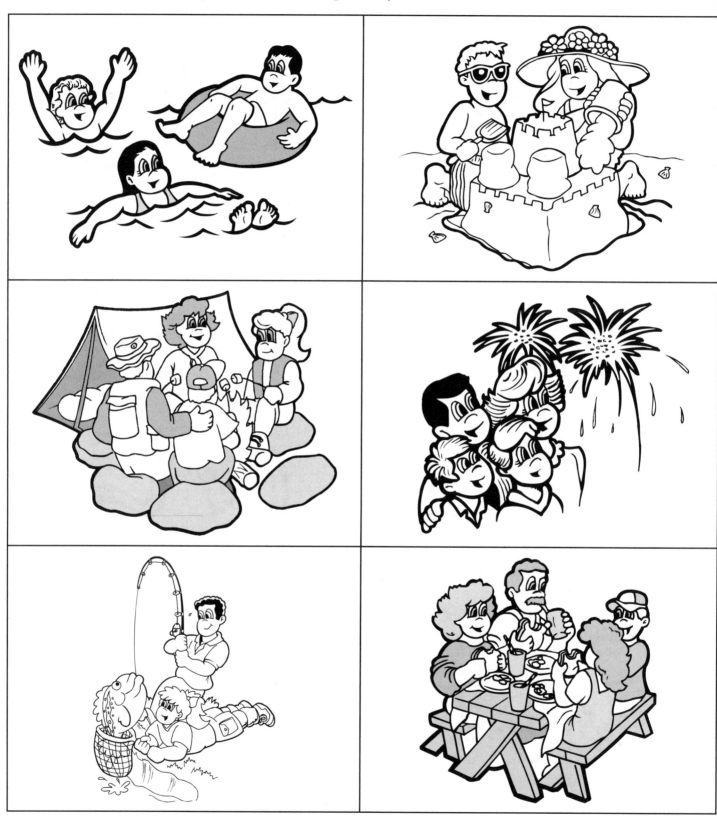

Name _____  Date _____

Speech-Language Pathologist                    Helper's Signature

#BK-272  Year-Round Literature  •  ©1999 Super Duper® Publications  •  1-800-277-8737  •  www.superduperinc.com

# Dinosaurs

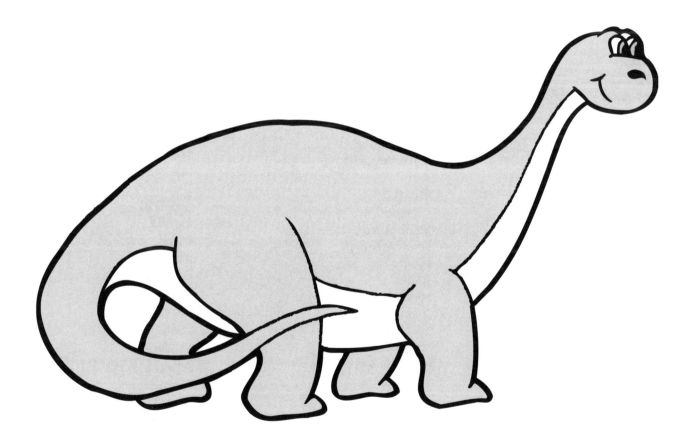

# Dinosaurs Articulation & Vocabulary Word Lists

These word lists are a good resource for articulation and/or vocabulary building activities.

## /r/ and /r/ blends

### Initial
reptile
run
raptor

### Medial
Allosaurus
Stegosaurus
Jurassic Period
Tyrannosaurus Rex
Ankylosaurus
Theropod
Pterodactyl

### Final
dinosaur
plant-eater
herbivore
meat-eater
carnivore
Phytosaur
Hadrosaur

### Blends
Brachiosaurus
Triceratops
prehistoric
predator
prey
Protoceratops
Brontosauraus
sharp teeth
sharp claws
footprint
Earth
warm-blooded
large
horns

## /s/ and /s/ blends

### Initial
scientist
site

### Medial
dinosaur
fossil
Jurassic Period

Tyrannosaurus Rex
Phytosaur
Brontosauraus

### Final
Allosaurus
Diplodocus
footprints
Ankylosaurus
plants
Albertosaurus
Megalosaurus
Protoceratops
Stegosaurus
Struthiosaurus
Tyrannosaurus Rex
Triceratops
Brachiosaurus
Allosaurus
Plateosaurus
Hadrosaurus
Carnosaurus
Styracosaurus

### Blends
skeleton
Spinosaurus
Struthiosaurus
skull
spine
spikes
species
Spinosaurus
Stegosaurus
Styracosaurus
scaly skin
skeleton
extinct
paleontologist
prehistoric
nest

## /z/

### Medial
museum

### Final
sharp claws
horns
bones
claws

eggs
legs

## /l/ and /l/ blends

### Initial
legs
long neck
large

### Medial
Allosaurus
paleontologist
scaly skin
skeleton
Megalosaurus
Woolly Mammoth
volcano

### Final
reptile
skull
tail

### Blends
fossil
sharp claws
plant-eater
cold-blooded
flying dinosaur
plants
Diplodocus
Anklyosaurus
Albertosaurus
Pterodactyl

## /k/ and /k/ blends

### Initial
carnivore
Camarasaurus
Compsognathus
Carnosaur
cave

### Medial
extinct
Jurassic Period

#BK-272  Year-Round Literature • ©1999 Super Duper® Publications • 1-800-277-8737 • www.superduperinc.com

# Dinosaurs Articulation & Vocabulary Word Lists (Cont.)

## /k/ and /k/ blends cont.

### Medial cont.
Brachiosaurus
excavation
Styracosaurus

### Final
prehistoric
walk
beak
long neck

### Blends
Ankylosaurus
sharp claws
scaly skin
skeleton
Kritosaurus
excavation
claw
skull
spikes
Tyrannosaurus Rex

## /g/ and /g/ blends

### Medial
Stegosaurus
Iguanodon
Megalosaurus

### Final
big
egg

### Blends
legs

## /th/

### Initial
The Age of the Dinosaur
Theropod
Therizinosaurus

### Medial
Ornithopoda
Struthiosaurus
Compsognathus

### Final
tooth
mouth
Earth
mammoth

## /sh/

### Initial
sharp teeth
sharp claws
Shunosaurus

### Medial
excavation

## /ch/

### Initial
Chasmosaurus
chew

## /m/ and /m/ blends

### Initial
Megalosaurus
meat-eater

### Medial
Camarasaurus
Chasmosaurus
mammoth

### Final
museum

### Blends
warm-blooded

## /p/ and /p/ blends

### Medial
reptile
Apatosaurus
Theropod
Ornithipoda

### Blends
plant eater
prehistoric
Plateosaurus
predator
prey
plants
Protoceratops
Diplodocus
Triceratops
footprints
Spinosaurus
spine
species
spikes
raptors
sharp

## /b/ and /b/ blends

### Initial
bones
beak
big

### Medial
herbivore

### Blends
Brachiosaurus
warm-blooded
cold-blooded
Fabrosaurus

## /f/ and /f/ blends

### Initial
fossil
footprints
Phytosaur
Fabrosaurus
foot

### Blends
flying dinosaur

## /v/

### Initial
volcano

### Medial
herbivore
carnivore
excavation

### Final
cave

# Vocabulary Pictures

**Instructions:** _____

_____

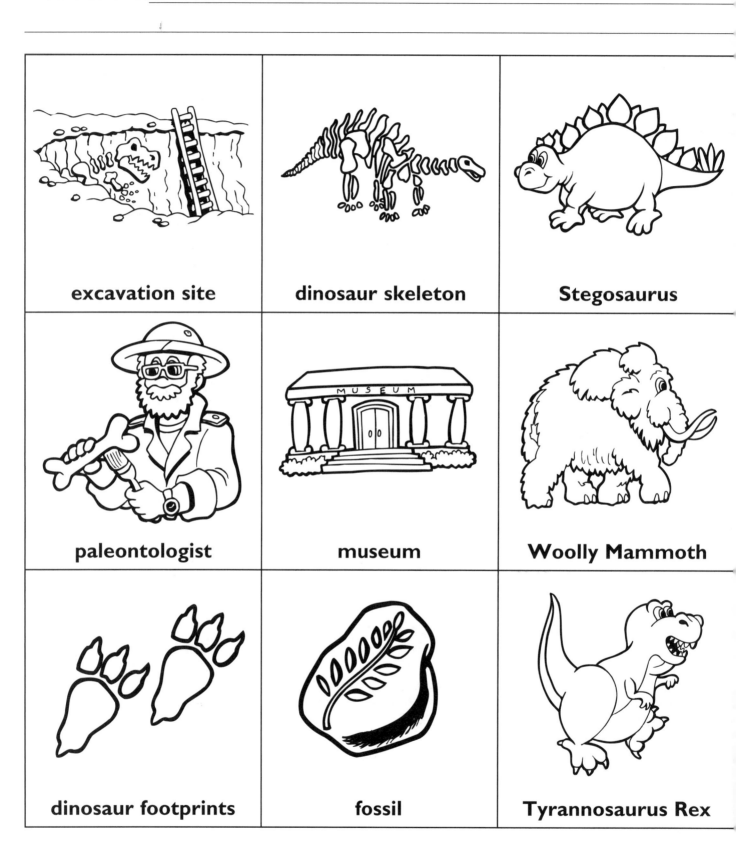

excavation site

dinosaur skeleton

Stegosaurus

paleontologist

museum

Woolly Mammoth

dinosaur footprints

fossil

Tyrannosaurus Rex

Name _____  Date _____

#BK-272  Year-Round Literature • ©1999 Super Duper® Publications • 1-800-277-8737 • www.superduperinc.com

# Vocabulary Pictures

Instructions: _____

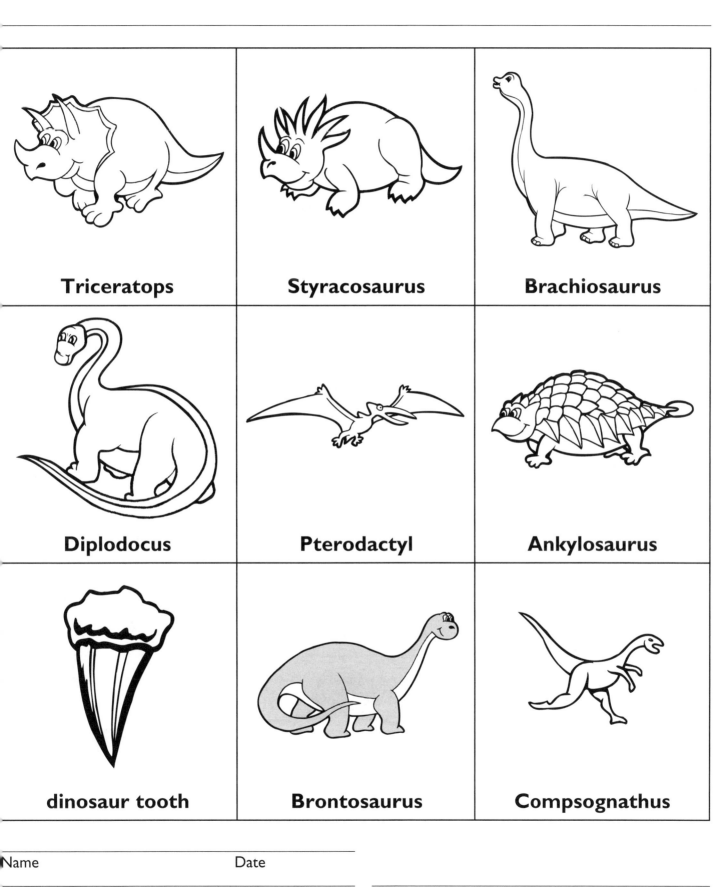

| | | |
|---|---|---|
| **Triceratops** | **Styracosaurus** | **Brachiosaurus** |
| **Diplodocus** | **Pterodactyl** | **Ankylosaurus** |
| **dinosaur tooth** | **Brontosaurus** | **Compsognathus** |

Name _____ Date _____

Speech-Language Pathologist _____ Helper's Signature _____

# Vocabulary Pictures

**Instructions:** _____

_____

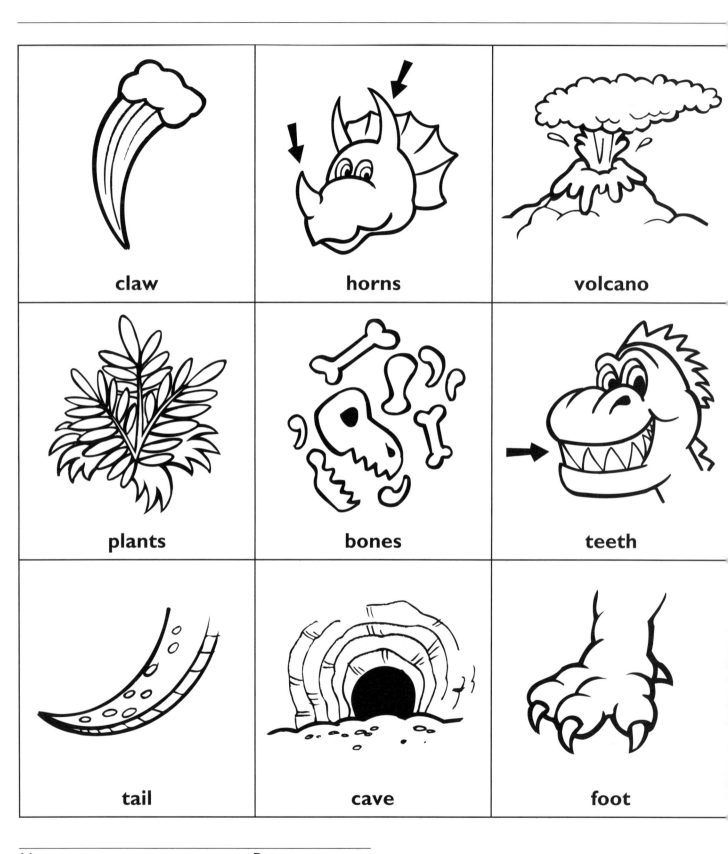

claw

horns

volcano

plants

bones

teeth

tail

cave

foot

Name _____   Date _____

Speech-Language Pathologist          Helper's Signature

#BK-272  Year-Round Literature  •  ©1999 Super Duper® Publications  •  1-800-277-8737  •  www.superduperinc.com

# Story Pattern

Name:

_____

_____

_____

_____

_____

_____

_____

_____

_____

_____

_____

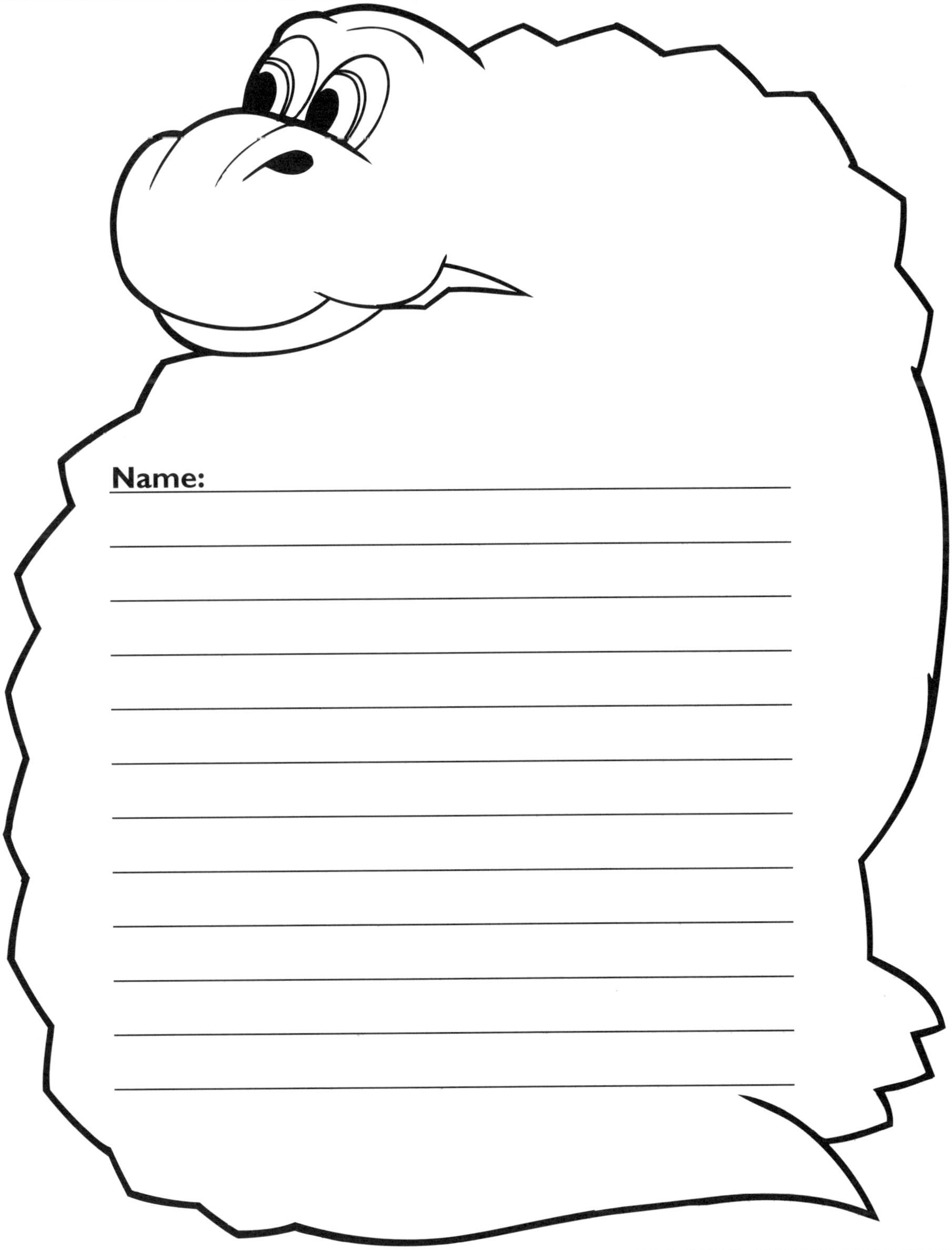

Name                                    Date

Speech-Language Pathologist                    Helper's Signature

#BK-272  Year-Round Literature  •  ©1999 Super Duper® Publications  •  1-800-277-8737  •  www.superduperinc.com

# Whatever Happened to the Dinosaurs?
## by Bernard Most

This book gives answers to the questions that many children have asked: "Whatever happened to the dinosaurs?" The author gives several amusing answers to the age-old question. The book ends by listing the many kinds of dinosaurs and asks the reader, "Do you know what happened to the dinosaurs?"

**Language Expansion:** The following questions can be used to address students' recall of this book or to expand upon concepts addressed in this book.

## Definition
1. What is a dinosaur?
2. What is a library?
3. What is a scientist?
4. What is a disguise?
5. What is hibernating?

## Function
1. What is a library used for?
2. What is a scientist used for?
3. What is a magician used for?
4. What is a disguise used for?
5. What is a hospital used for?

## Category
1. Name three kinds of dinosaurs.
2. Name three things you can do at a library.
3. Name three planets.
4. Name three places for a vacation.
5. Name three things that may have happened to the dinosaurs.

## Description
1. Tell me three things about a dinosaur.
2. Tell me three things you can read in a library.
3. Tell me three people you can find in a hospital.
4. Tell me three things about a jungle.
5. Tell me three things about a vacation.

## Vocabulary
Make a sentence using the following words.
1. dinosaur
2. scientist
3. disguise
4. vacation
5. hibernating

## Rhyming
Name a rhyming word for each word below
1. meat
2. know
3. tooth
4. claw
5. scream

## Sequencing
As your students sequence the events in this story, use this list as a guide.

1. The children wonder if the dinosaurs went to another planet.
2. The children wonder if a magician made the dinosaurs disappear.
3. The children wonder if the dinosaurs are wearing disguises.
4. The children wonder if the dinosaurs are in the hospital or in jail.
5. The children wonder if the dinosaurs are lost in the jungle or mistaken for dragons.
6. The children wonder if the pirates stole the dinosaurs or if the dinosaurs are living underground.
7. The children wonder if the dinosaurs go on vacation or only come out at night.
8. The children wonder if there was no room for the dinosaurs on Noah's ark. Are they hibernating or did they shrink so we can't see them?
9. The children wonder if the dinosaurs are on the North Pole or underwater.
10. The children wonder if the dinosaurs had a shortage of food or are playing hide-and-seek.

#BK-272 Year-Round Literature • ©1999 Super Duper® Publications • 1-800-277-8737 • www.superduperinc.com

# I Met a Dinosaur
## by Jan Wahl

This is a book about a little girl who imagines that she sees dinosaurs in places such as a gas station, a park, a lake, and several other locations. Her trip to the museum has peeked her interest about dinosaurs and her imagination is hard at work. The story ends with a page that names and describes several types of dinosaurs.

---

**Language Expansion:** The following questions can be used to address students' recall of this book

## Definition
1. What is a dinosaur?
2. What is a museum?
3. What is a gas pump?
4. What is a shed?
5. What is fog?

## Function
1. What is a museum for?
2. What is a road used for?
3. What is a gas station used for?
4. What is a railroad track used for?
5. What is a kite used for?

## Category
1. Name three kinds of dinosaurs.
2. Name three things you might see at a museum.
3. Name three things to drink.
4. Name the days of the week.
5. Name three places the little girl thought that she saw the dinosaur.

## Description
1. Tell me three things about dinosaurs.
2. Tell me three things about a museum.
3. Tell me three things about a gas station.
4. Tell me three things about a railroad track.
5. Tell me three things about a kite.

## Vocabulary
Make a sentence using the following words.
1. dinosaur
2. museum
3. fog
4. gas pump
5. kite

## Rhyming
Name a rhyming word for each word below.
1. shed
2. pump
3. fog
4. kite
5. drink

---

## Sequencing
As your students sequence the events in this story, use this list as a guide.

1. A little girl meets a dinosaur in the museum and she imagines what the dinosaurs would do.
2. On Tuesday night, a Stegosaurus was at play at the gas station.
3. On Wednesday night, a Dimetrodon was behind the shed looking to be fed.
4. On Thursday night, a Triceratops stood near a railroad track.
5. On Friday night, an Iguanadon was at the lake.
6. On Saturday night, a Tyrannosaurus was hiding in the trees.
7. On Sunday night, a Pterodactyl was flying in the sky.

# Can I Have a Stegosaurus Mom? Can I? Please!?
## by Lois G. Grambling

This amusing book is about a boy who wants a Stegosaurus for a pet. He tries to convince his mother to allow him to have a Stegosaurus by telling her about all of the things that a Stegosaurus could do for him. Finally, the little boy decides that if he can't have a Stegosaurus, maybe he could have a Tyrannosaurus Rex.

**Language Expansion:** The following questions can be used to address students' recall of this book or to expand upon concepts addressed in this book.

## Definition
1. What is a Stegosaurus?
2. What is a parade?
3. What is a field trip?
4. What is a tug of war?
5. What is a mascot?

## Function
1. What is the boy's Stegosaurus used for in this story?
2. What is summer camp for?
3. What is an egg used for?
4. What is a plate used for?
5. What is a drum major used for?

## Category
1. Name three things you can do with a Stegosaurus.
2. Name three places that are big enough that a boy could hide a Stegosaurus.
3. Name three things that a dinosaur might like to eat.
4. Name three parts of a dinosaur.
5. Name three things you can see in a parade.

## Description
1. Tell me three things about a Stegosaurus
2. Tell me three things about a parade.
3. Tell me three things about the North Pole.
4. Tell me three things about the egg at the end of the story.
5. Tell me three things about a football game.

## Vocabulary
Make a sentence using the following words.
1. Stegosaurus
2. parade
3. tail
4. Halloween
5. bleachers

## Rhyming
Name a rhyming word for each word below
1. camp
2. plate
3. drum
4. game
5. tail

## Sequencing
As your students sequence the events in this story, use this list as a guide.
1. The little boy would like to have a Stegosaurus for a pet.
2. The little boy says a Stegosaurus could sleep in his bed at night and pounce on scary monsters.
3. The little boy says a Stegosaurus could eat all of his yucky vegetables or take his class on a field trip if they missed the bus.
4. The little boy says a Stegosaurus could give him the best view of a parade, be the mascot for his peewee football team, or take him to the North Pole to tell Santa what he left off his Christmas list.
5. The little boy decides that if he can't have a Stegosaurus that maybe his mom would let him have a Tyrannosaurus Rex.

#BK-272 Year-Round Literature • ©1999 Super Duper® Publications • 1-800-277-8737 • www.superduperinc.com

# Dinosaurs Articulation and Language Games

(The following games can be used with the articulation and vocabulary word list or the literature language questions.)

## Tyrannosaurus Rex Puzzle Game

Photocopy, color, laminate, and cut out the T-Rex puzzle (page 94) for each student. Put each puzzle into a separate envelope. When playing, give each student a puzzle with all of the pieces facedown. After a student makes a sentence with a dinosaur word containing his/her sound or answers a dinosaur language question, the student may turn over one piece of his/her puzzle. The object is for each student to have his/her puzzle completely together by the end of class.

### Language Extension

After completing the puzzle, allow each student to describe one particular part of the T-Rex. Talk about what the real T-Rexes looked like, what it might have sounded like, etc.

## Help the Paleontologist Find the Bones Game

Make one copy of the paleontologist dig game board (page 95) for each student. Color and laminate each game board. Cut out and laminate the direction cards. The object of the game is to help the paleontologist get to the dinosaur bones. After a student makes a sentence with a dinosaur word containing his/her sound or answers a dinosaur language question, the student may choose a direction card. The direction card will tell the student to move forward a certain number of steps, backward a certain number of steps, or to remain in place. The student who gets to the bones is the winner of the game.

### Language Extension

After completing the game, ask the students to brainstorm the things they might see on a paleontologist dig. Then, discuss what you might take on a paleontologist dig and why you might take the items.

## Dinosaur Matching Game

Make two copies of the dinosaur matching game (page 96). Color the dinosaurs, cut them apart, and laminate them. Lay the cards facedown and allow each student to turn over two cards. If the cards don't match, the student must choose one of the cards to name and describe using good speech and language and then put both cards facedown. If the cards match, the student must tell about the dinosaur by naming it and then describing it using good speech and language. Then, the student may keep the matching pair. Continue taking turns until all of the dinosaurs have been matched. The student with the most matches is the winner.

### Team Approach

In order to win the game, the team must be able to match all of the dinosaurs by the end of the therapy session.

## Dinosaur Egg Game

Photocopy the dinosaur eggs (page 97) and one dinosaur nest (page 98) for each student. Color, cut out, and laminate the eggs and nest. Give each student a nest to place on the table. Put all of the dinosaur egg cards facedown in a pile on the table. After a student makes a sentence with a dinosaur word containing his/her sound or answers a dinosaur language question, the student may choose one card from the pile. If the card shows a whole dinosaur egg, the student puts it in his/her nest. If the card shows a dinosaur egg cracked open, the student returns the card to the pile. The student with the most dinosaur eggs at the end is the winner, or each student is a winner if he/she has at least five dinosaur eggs in his/her basket.

### Language Extension

Talk about dinosaur eggs, different types of dinosaurs, and when the dinosaurs lived.

## Dinosaur Game

Photocopy, color, cut out, and laminate the dinosaurs (page 99). Turn the cards facedown. After a student makes a sentence with a dinosaur word containing his/her sound or answers a dinosaur language question, the student chooses one dinosaur card. If the dinosaur has directions, the student must follow the directions. If the dinosaur is blank, the student may keep the dinosaur. The student with the most dinosaurs at the end of the game is the winner.

### Team Approach

In order to win the game, the team must get a designated number of dinosaurs. For example, the team must have 15 dinosaurs by the end of class to win.

# T-Rex Puzzle Game

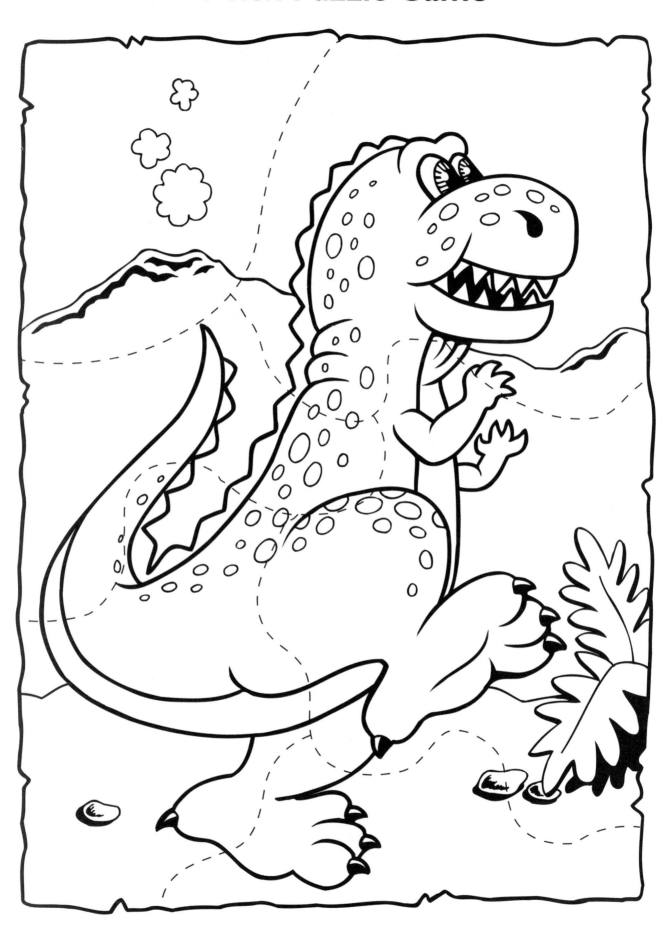

#BK-272   Year-Round Literature   •   ©1999 Super Duper® Publications   •   1-800-277-8737   •   www.superduperinc.com

# Help the Paleontologist Find the Bones.

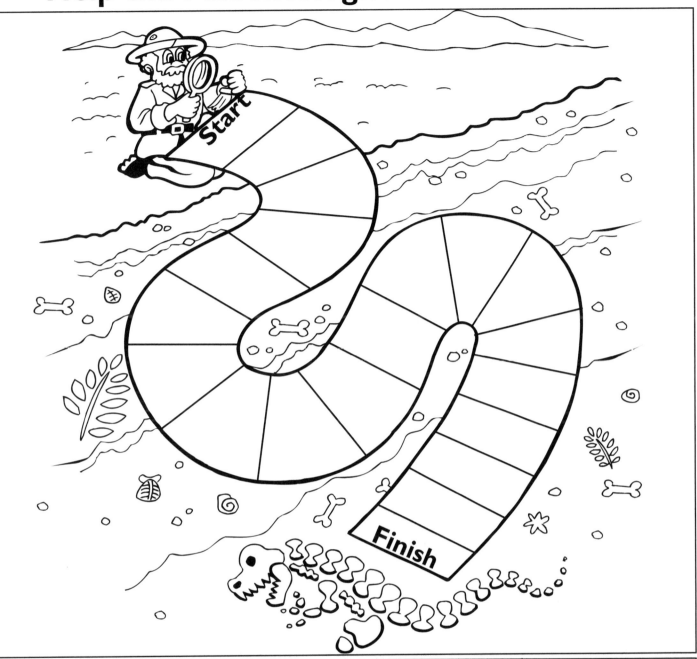

| Found a fossil! Go forward 3 steps. | Shovel broke. Go backward 3 steps. | Packed your supplies well. Go forward 2 steps. | You're digging well. Go forward 1 step. |
|---|---|---|---|
| Sandstorm blows through. Go backward 2 steps. | It is starting to rain. Go backward 1 step. | Hit a rock while digging. Stay where you are. | You brought a map. Go forward 1 step. |

# Dinosaur Matching Game

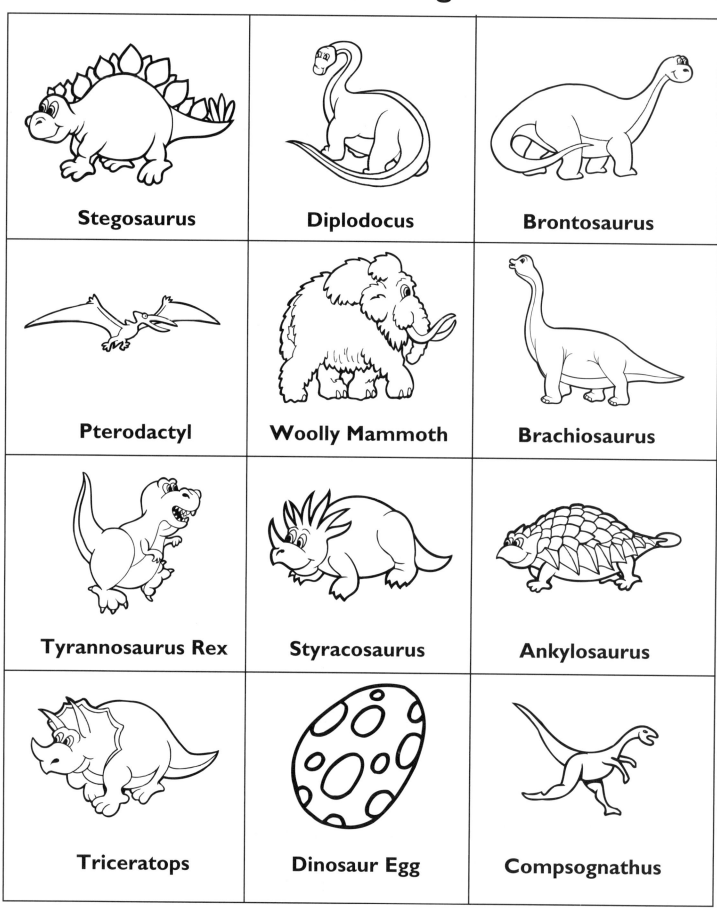

Stegosaurus

Diplodocus

Brontosaurus

Pterodactyl

Woolly Mammoth

Brachiosaurus

Tyrannosaurus Rex

Styracosaurus

Ankylosaurus

Triceratops

Dinosaur Egg

Compsognathus

#BK-272  Year-Round Literature  •  ©1999 Super Duper® Publications  •  1-800-277-8737  •  www.superduperinc.com

# Dinosaur Egg Game

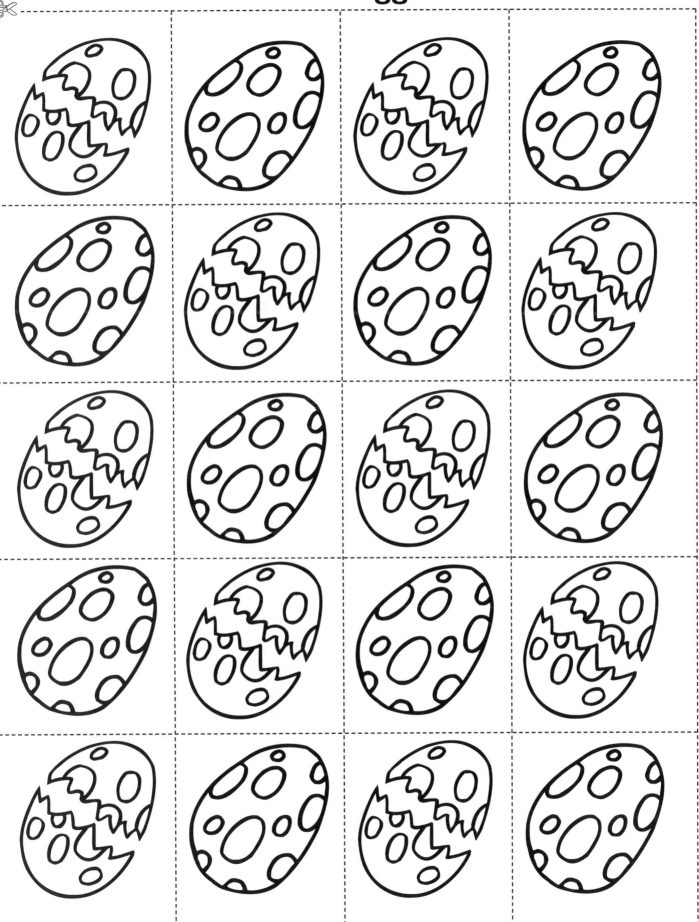

# Dinosaur Egg Game

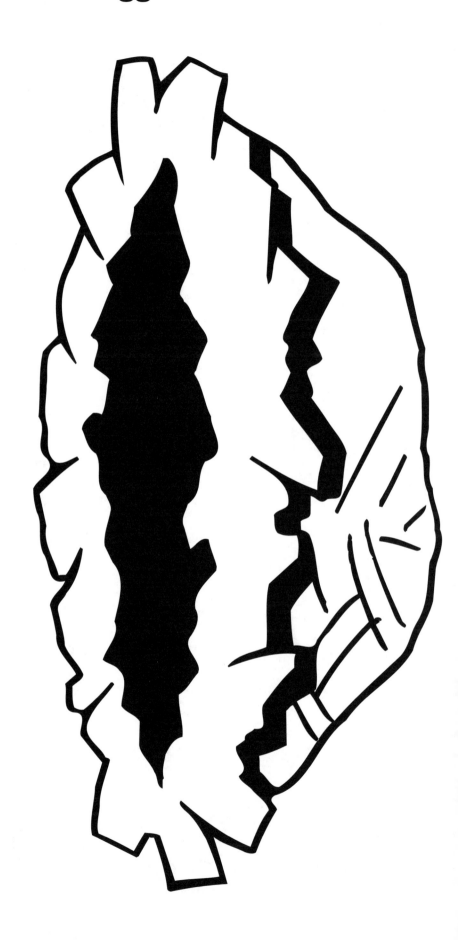

#BK-272  Year-Round Literature  •  ©1999 Super Duper® Publications  •  1-800-277-8737  •  www.superduperinc.com

# Dinosaur Game

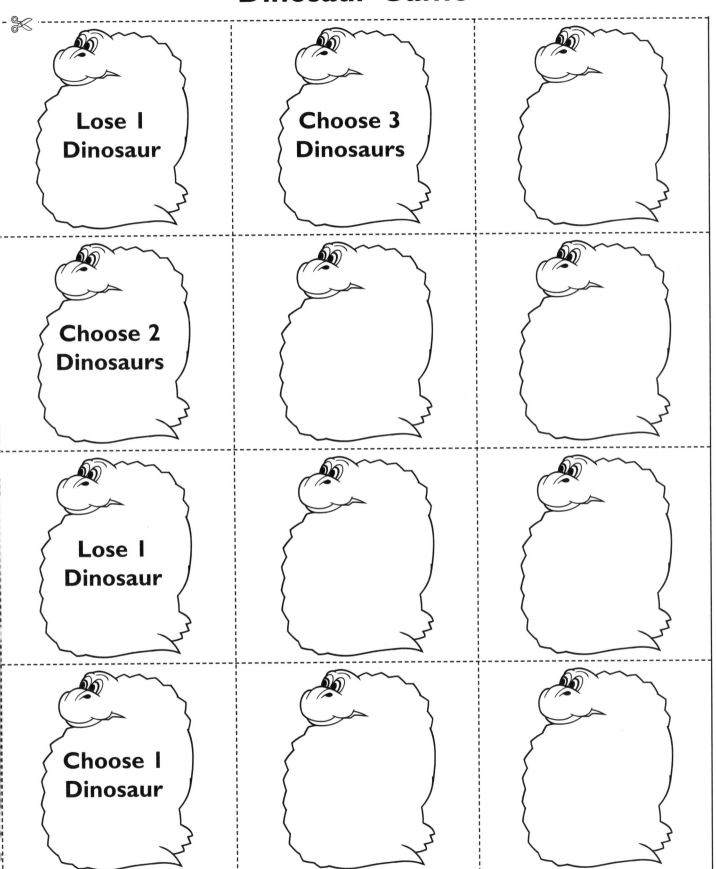

Lose 1
Dinosaur

Choose 3
Dinosaurs

Choose 2
Dinosaurs

Lose 1
Dinosaur

Choose 1
Dinosaur

# Dino-mite Speech

Write a _____in each spot of the dinosaur.
Then, make a sentence with each word out loud using your good speech.

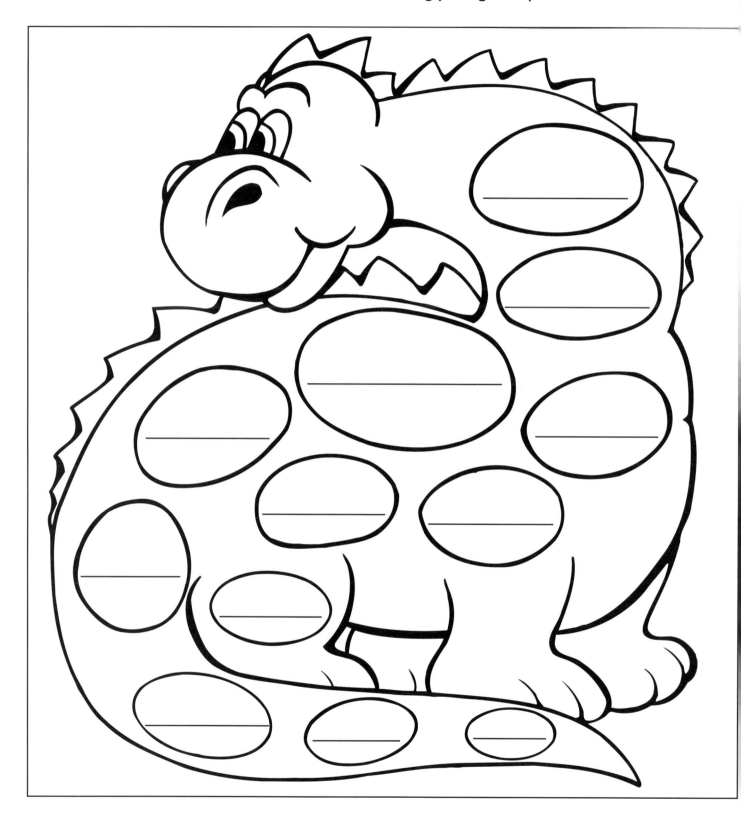

Name _____     Date _____

Speech-Language Pathologist _____     Helper's Signature _____

#BK-272  Year-Round Literature  •  ©1999 Super Duper® Publications  •  1-800-277-8737  •  www.superduperinc.com

# Dinosaur Matching

Read each description.  Then, see if you can find the picture that matches each description. Draw a line from the description to the matching picture.

| | |
|---|---|
| A large reptile that lived on Earth many years ago and then became extinct. | |
| The sharp objects in the jaw that dinosaurs used to eat meat or plants. | |
| A person who studies fossils and things that lived long ago. | |
| Dinosaurs laid these and when they hatched, there would be a baby dinosaur. | |
| The remains of an animal or plant that have been preserved in the soil or rock. | |

Name _____  Date _____

Speech-Language Pathologist _____  Helper's Signature _____

# Parts of a Dinosaur

Can you name each part of the dinosaur?  Cut out the words below and put them in the correct place.

| Head | Teeth | Neck | Feet | Tail | Horns | Spine | Forelimb | Hindlimb |
|------|-------|------|------|------|-------|-------|----------|----------|

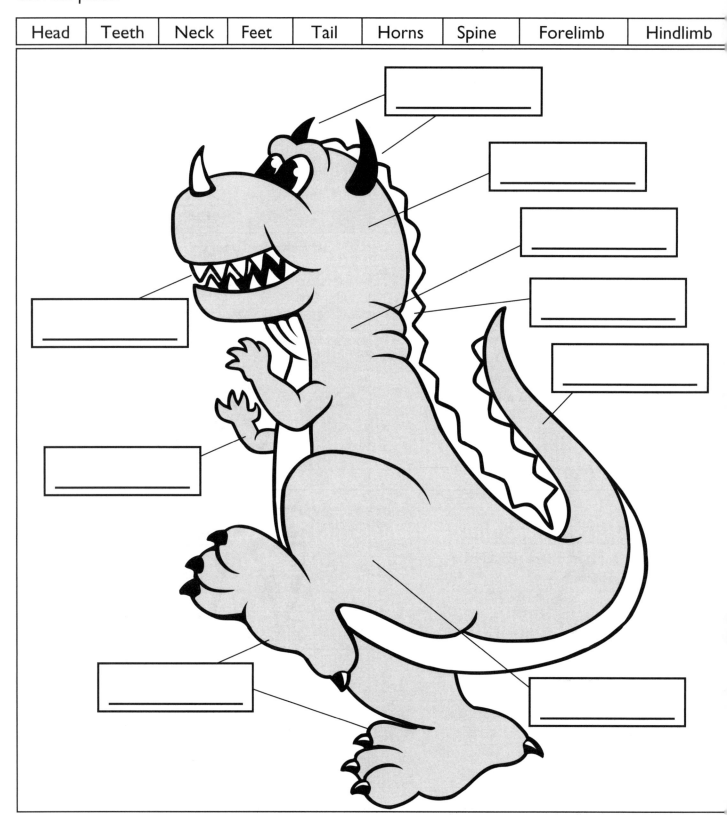

Name _____          Date _____

_____

Speech-Language Pathologist                    Helper's Signature

#BK-272  Year-Round Literature  •  ©1999 Super Duper® Publications  •  1-800-277-8737  •  www.superduperinc.com

# Circus

# Circus Articulation & Vocabulary Word Lists

These word lists are a good resource for articulation and/or vocabulary building activities.

## /r/ and /r/ blends

### Initial
rings
red nose
rope

### Medial
daredevil
aerialist
giraffe
parade
colorful costumes
somersault

### Final
high wire
bear
tiger
lion tamer
panther
vendor
juggler
ringmaster

### Blends
trapeze
trampoline
pretzels
drinks
"Greatest Show on Earth"
train
tricks
acrobat
popcorn
perform
horse
circus
circus tent
circus stars
Barnum and Bailey
riders
Ringling Brothers

## /s/ and /s/ blends

### Initial
soda
seal

### Medial
circus tent

horses
unicycle
bicycle
somersault

### Final
circus
audience
dance
peanuts
balance
acts
tricks
lights

### Blends
stage
circus stars
stilts
spotlight
costume
aerialist
ring master
"Greatest Show on Earth"
artist

## /z/

### Initial
zebra

### Medial
music

### Final
funny faces
red nose
trapeze
dogs
animals
ponies
hot dogs
Ringling Brothers
feathers
riders
applause
circus stars

## /l/ and /l/ blends

### Initial
laugh
lion
lion tamer
lights
llama
leopard
lady

### Medial
elephant
aerialist
spotlight
trampoline
balloons
balance
hula hoop
Barnum and Bailey

### Final
daredevil
seal
camel
pole

### Blends
clowns
applause
flip
clown make-up
juggler
stilts
Ringling Brothers
juggler
unicycle
bicycle
pretzel

## /k/ and /k/ blends

### Initial
costume
cotton candy
cage
camel

#BK-272 Year-Round Literature • ©1999 Super Duper® Publications • 1-800-277-8737 • www.superduperinc.com

# Circus Articulation & Vocabulary Word Lists (Cont.)

## /k/ and /k/ blends cont.

### Medial
circus
monkey
circus tent
popcorn
ticket
circus stars

### Final
music
horseback

### Blends
clown
clown make-up
clap
acrobat
unicycle
bicycle
drinks
acts
tricks

## /g/

### Medial
tiger
big top

### Final
dog
hot dog
wig

### Blends
"Greatest Show on Earth"
juggle
juggler

## /th/ and /th/ blends

### Medial
Ringling Brothers
feathers
panther

### Final
lion's teeth
lion's mouth
"Greatest Show on Earth"
booth

### Blends
three-ring circus

## /sh/

### Initial
shoulders
show

### Final
crash

## /m/

### Initial
monkey
music
make-up

### Medial
ring master
lion tamer
llama
somersault

### Final
costume
perform
trampoline

### Blends
camel
animal

## /p/ and /p/ blends

### Initial
ponies
popcorn
peanuts
perform
parade
pole

### Medial
trapeze
leopard

### Final
tightrope
whip
clown make-up

Big Top
flip
hulahoop
hoop

### Blends
pretzels
spotlight
applause
trampoline

## /b/ and /b/ blends

### nitial
bear
bicycle
balloon
balance
Barnum
Bailey
band
Big Top
bow
booth

### Blends
Ringling Brothers
zebra

## /f/ and /f/ blends

### Initial
funny faces
fun

### Medial
elephant

### Final
laugh

### Blends
flip

## /v/ and /v/ blends

### Initial
vendor

### Blends
daredevil

# Vocabulary Pictures

**Instructions:** _____

_____

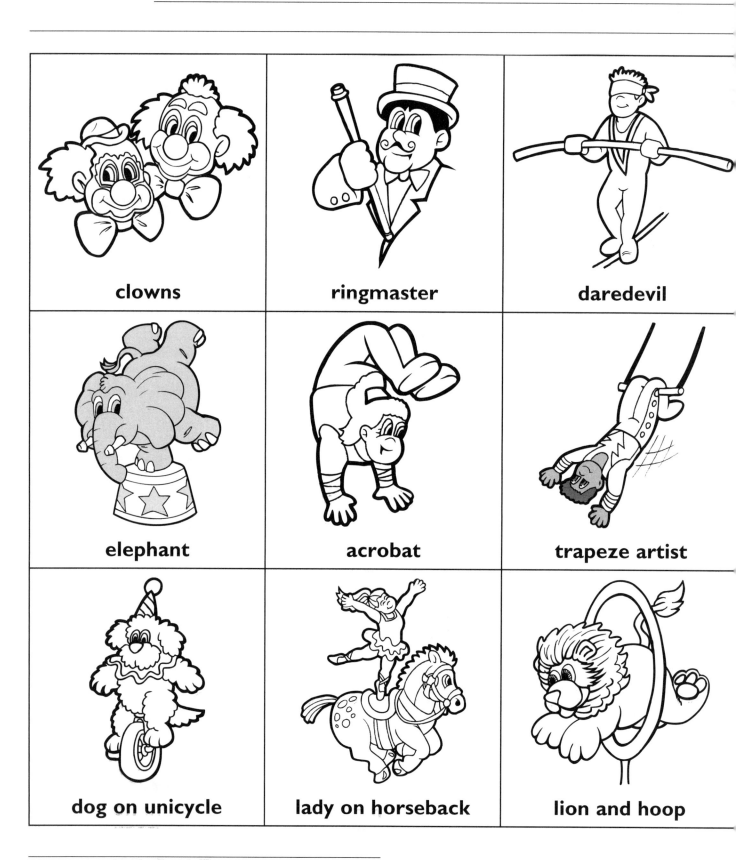

| | | |
|---|---|---|
| **clowns** | **ringmaster** | **daredevil** |
| **elephant** | **acrobat** | **trapeze artist** |
| **dog on unicycle** | **lady on horseback** | **lion and hoop** |

Name _____ Date _____

Speech-Language Pathologist      Helper's Signature

#BK-272 Year-Round Literature • ©1999 Super Duper® Publications • 1-800-277-8737 • www.superduperinc.com

# Vocabulary Pictures

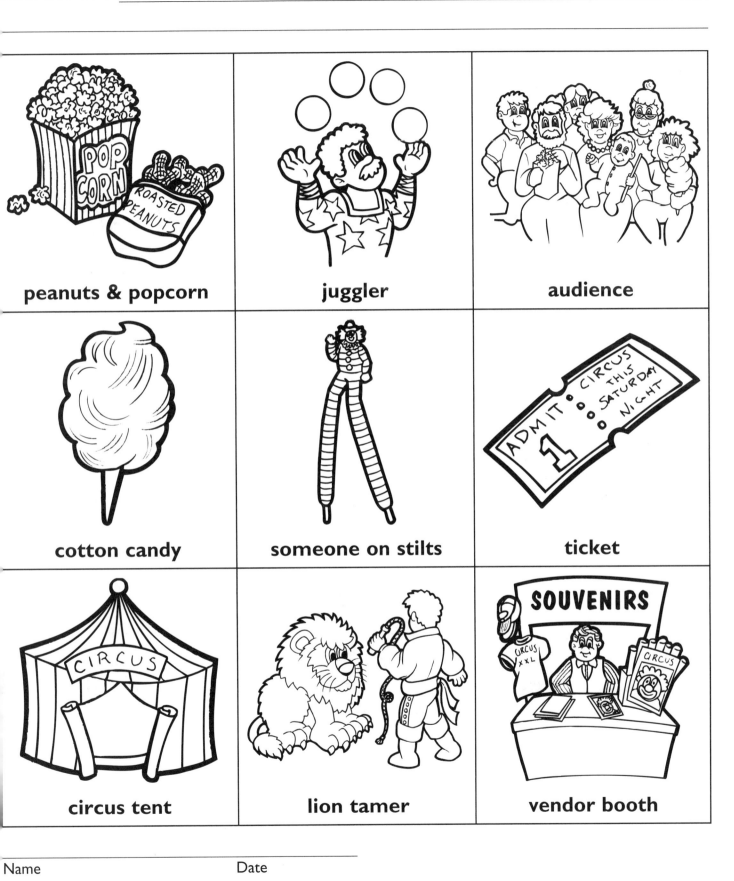

peanuts & popcorn

juggler

audience

cotton candy

someone on stilts

ticket

circus tent

lion tamer

vendor booth

Name _____ Date _____

Speech-Language Pathologist                    Helper's Signature

# Vocabulary Pictures

**Instructions:** _____

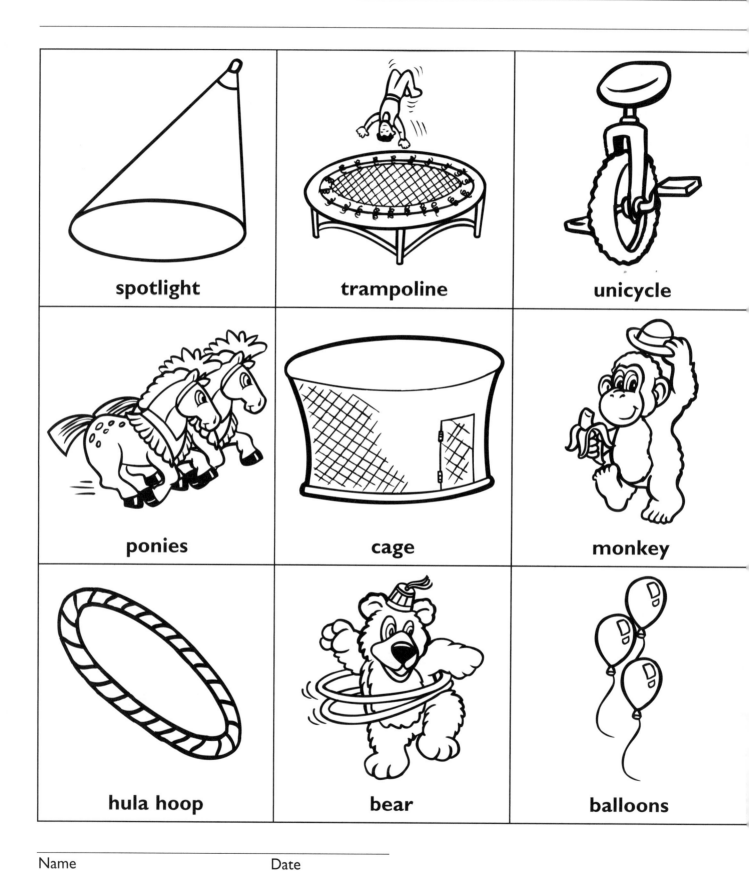

| | | |
|---|---|---|
| spotlight | trampoline | unicycle |
| ponies | cage | monkey |
| hula hoop | bear | balloons |

Name _____ Date _____

# Story Pattern

**Name:** _____

_____

_____

_____

_____

_____

_____

_____

_____

_____

_____

_____

_____

_____

_____

_____

_____

_____

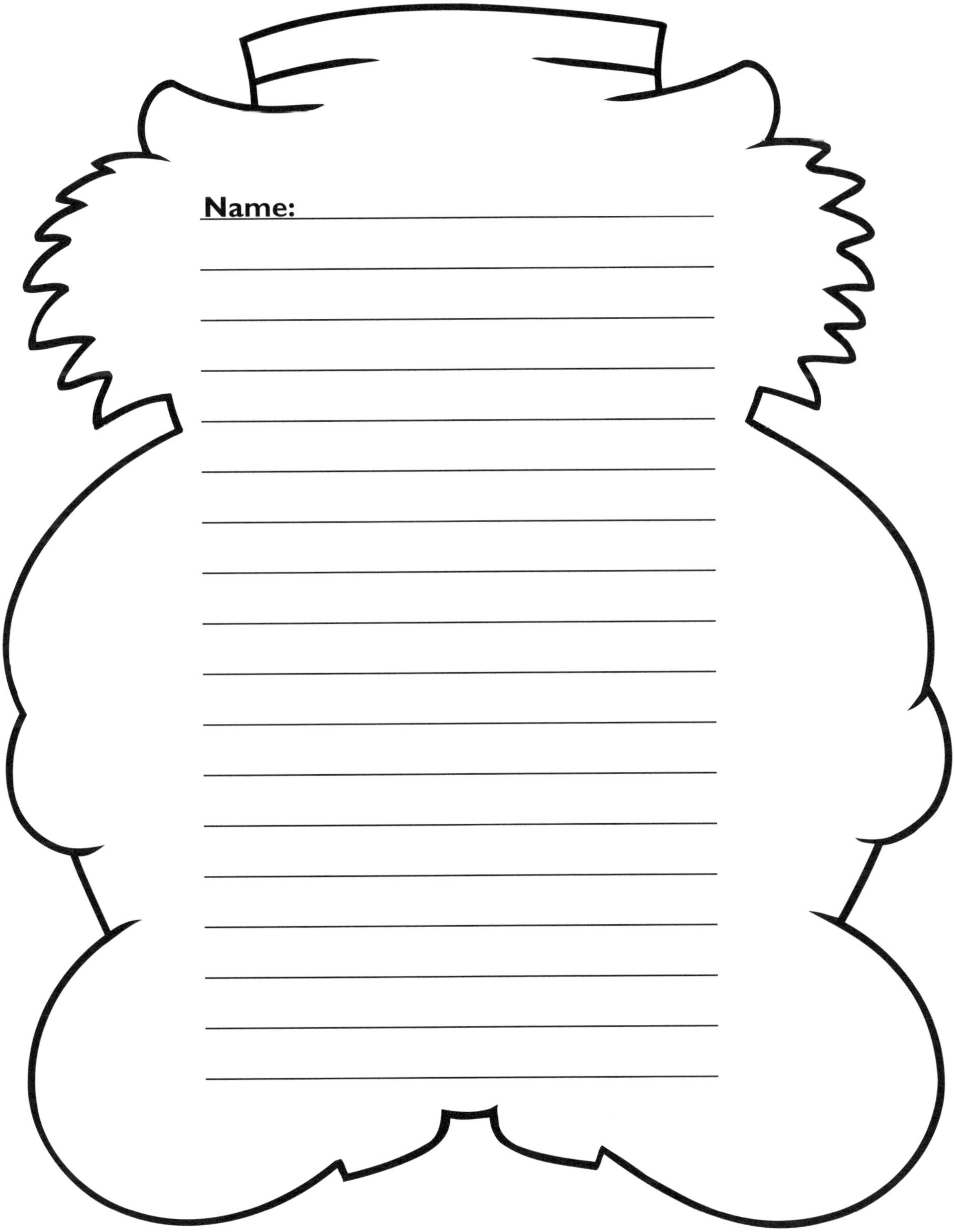

Name _____     Date _____

Speech-Language Pathologist _____     Helper's Signature _____

# Olivia Saves the Circus
## by Ian Falconer

This is a fun story about Olivia, the pig. She goes to school and is asked to tell the class about her vacation. She makes up a story about how her mother took her to the circus. But, when they got there, all of the circus people were sick and so she had to perform the entire show.

**Language Expansion:** The following questions can be used to address students' recall of this book or to expand upon concepts addressed in this book.

## Definition
1. What is a school?
2. What is a uniform?
3. What is an audience?
4. What is a unicycle?
5. What is a trampoline?

## Function
1. What is breakfast for?
2. What is a uniform for?
3. What is an audience for?
4. What is a unicycle for?
5. What is a lion tamer for?

## Category
1. Name three things you can have for breakfast.
2. Name three things you see at a circus.
3. Name three things Olivia did at the circus.
4. Name three things Olivia wore to school.
5. Name three things in Olivia's bedroom.

## Description
1. Tell me three things about Olivia.
2. Tell me three things about Olivia's uniform.
3. Tell me three things about Olivia's family.
4. Tell me three things about the circus.
5. Tell me three things about Olivia's bedroom.

## Vocabulary
Make a sentence using the following words.
1. accessorize
2. vacation
3. infection
4. stilts
5. famous

## Rhyming
Name a rhyming word for each word below.
1. nice
2. wear
3. tell
4. sick
5. night

## Sequencing
As your students sequence the events in this story, use this list as a guide.
1. Olivia gets up and helps her mother make pancakes before school.
2. Olivia puts on her uniform and goes to school.
3. At school, it is Olivia's turn to tell the class about her vacation.
4. She tells them about going to the circus and all of the performers are sick.
5. Olivia takes the place of the performers at the circus.
6. Olivia goes home and at bedtime her mother reminds her not to jump on her bed.
7. But Olivia jumps and her mother comes to tell her to stop, asking her if she is the "Queen of the Trampoline."

#BK-272 Year-Round Literature • ©1999 Super Duper® Publications • 1-800-277-8737 • www.superduperinc.com

# The Circus Surprise
## by Ralph Fletcher

Nick's parents always have a special plan for his birthday. This year they are all going to the circus. He is enjoying the circus, but he gets lost. A friendly clown on stilts helps Nick find his parents. What a fun birthday for Nick!

**Language Expansion:** The following questions can be used to address students' recall of this book or to expand upon concepts addressed in this book.

## Definition
1. What is a birthday?
2. What is a circus?
3. What is cotton candy?
4. What are stilts?
5. What is a ladder?

## Function
1. What is a trapeze for?
2. What is a cage for?
3. What is a cotton candy machine for?
4. What are stilts for?
5. What is a ladder for?

## Category
1. Name three things you see at the circus.
2. Name three things Nick did at the circus.
3. Name three animals that are in the circus.
4. Name three things a clown might do in the circus.
5. Name three things a clown might wear.

## Description
1. Tell me three things about Nick.
2. Tell me three things about the circus.
3. Tell me three things about cotton candy.
4. Tell me three things about a lion.
5. Tell me three things about a clown.

## Vocabulary
Make a sentence using the following words.
1. trapeze
2. muscles
3. cage
4. stilts
5. ladder

## Rhyming
Name a rhyming word for each word below.
1. air
2. place
3. lips
4. ants

## Sequencing
As your students sequence the events in this story, use this list as a guide.
1. Nick goes to the circus with his mom and dad for his birthday.
2. He enjoys seeing everything and stops at the cotton candy machine.
3. Nick gets lost and is frightened.
4. A friendly clown finds Nick.
5. The clown helps Nick find his parents.

# The 12 Circus Rings
## by Seymour Chwast

A little boy and his sister go to a circus that has 12 rings of exciting acts. The acts range from a daredevil on a high wire to animals doing tricks. The bright and colorful illustrations show all of the fun things that go on at the circus.

---

**Language Expansion:** The following questions can be used to address students' recall of this book or to expand upon concepts addressed in this book.

## Definition
1. What is a circus ring?
2. What is a high wire?
3. What is an elephant?
4. What is juggling?
5. What is an acrobat?

## Function
1. How is a high wire used?
2. How is a clown used?
3. How is a horse used?
4. How is a juggler used?
5. How is an elephant used?

## Category
1. Name three acts in the circus.
2. Name three animals in the circus.
3. Name three people in the circus.
4. Name three things you can leap over.
5. Name three things you could juggle.

## Description
1. Tell me three things about the circus.
2. Tell me three things about a clown.
3. Tell me three things about an aerialist.
4. Tell me three things about the circus ring.
5. Tell me three things about a juggler.

## Vocabulary
Make a sentence using the following words.
1. acrobat
2. juggle
3. monkey
4. horseback rider
5. laughing

## Rhyming
Name a rhyming word for each word below.
1. wire
2. ring
3. high
4. leap
5. sister

---

## Sequencing
As your students sequence the events in this story, use this list as a guide.

1. In the first circus ring there is a daredevil on a high wire.
2. In the second circus ring there are two elephants on a high wire.
3. In the third circus ring there are three monkeys playing.
4. In the fourth circus ring there are four aerialists zooming.
5. In the fifth circus ring there are five dogs barking.
6. In the sixth circus ring there are six acrobats.
7. In the seventh circus ring there are seven clowns clowning.
8. In the eighth circus ring there are eight bears performing.
9. In the ninth circus ring there are nine jugglers juggling.
10. In the tenth circus ring there are ten leapers leaping.
11. In the eleventh circus ring there are eleven horseback riders.
12. In the twelfth circus ring there are twelve animals laughing.

#BK-272 Year-Round Literature • ©1999 Super Duper® Publications • 1-800-277-8737 • www.superduperinc.com

# Circus Articulation and Language Games

(The following games can be used with the articulation and vocabulary word list or the literature language questions.)

## Decorate the Clown Game

Photocopy, color, and laminate the following game board (page 114). Then, photocopy the following student sheet (page 115) for each student. (You can photocopy front and back to save paper and use the back side with the next therapy group.) Make a game die using a penny. Put a piece of masking tape on both sides and write a "2" on one side and a "3" on the other side with permanent ink.

Discuss the different parts of the clown on the game board and tell the class that the goal is for each student to get each part in order to complete the clown on the student sheet. Then, give each child a student sheet and a pencil. After a student makes a sentence with a circus word containing his/her sound or answers a circus language question, the student may flip the penny die, move the allotted spaces around the game board, and then draw the clown part on the student sheet.

### Language Extension

After completing the clown, ask the student to name the parts and tell the purpose of each part.

## Circus Matching Game

Photocopy two copies of the circus objects (page 116). Color the circus items, cut them apart, and laminate them. Place the cards facedown and allow each student to turn over two cards. If the cards don't match, the student must choose one of the cards to name and describe using good speech and language and then put both cards facedown. If the cards match, the student must tell about the circus item by naming it and then describing it using good speech and language. Then, the student may keep the matching pair. Continue taking turns until all of the circus items have been matched. The student with the most matches is the winner.

### Team Approach

In order to win the game, the team must be able to match all of the circus items by the end of the therapy session.

## Ringmaster Game

Photocopy, color, cut out, and laminate the ringmasters (page 117). Turn the cards facedown. After a student makes a sentence with a circus word containing his/her sound or answers a circus language question, the student chooses one ringmaster card. If the ringmaster has directions, the student must follow the directions. If the ringmaster is blank, the student may keep the ringmaster. The student with the most ringmasters at the end of the game is the winner.

### Team Approach

In order to win the game, the team must receive a designated number of ringmasters. For example, the team must have 15 ringmasters by the end of class to win.

## Barrier Game

Color and laminate the circus scenes (pages 118 and 120). Color, cut out, and laminate items (page 119). Separate the students using a tall box or therapy mirror. Give one team a completed scene. Give the other team the empty scene and objects. The team with the completed scene must describe to the other team where each object should be placed. The team placing objects is allowed to ask three questions to ensure proper placement. The object is for the team with the empty scene and objects to re-create the completed scene of the other team. The game is ideal for students working on language and listening skills or for those students who are at the sentence or conversation level of articulation therapy.

## Where's the Circus? Game

Make one copy of the "Where's the Circus?" game board (page 121) for each student. Color, cut out, and laminate each game board and direction cards. The object of the game is to get the people to the circus. After a student makes a sentence with a circus word containing his/her sound or answers a circus language question, the student may choose a direction card. The direction card will tell the student to move forward a certain number of steps, backward a certain number of steps, or to remain in place. The student who gets to the circus first is the winner of the game.

### Language Extension

After completing the game, ask the students to brainstorm the things they might see at the circus. Then, discuss what you might eat or drink at the circus.

# Decorate the Clown Board Game

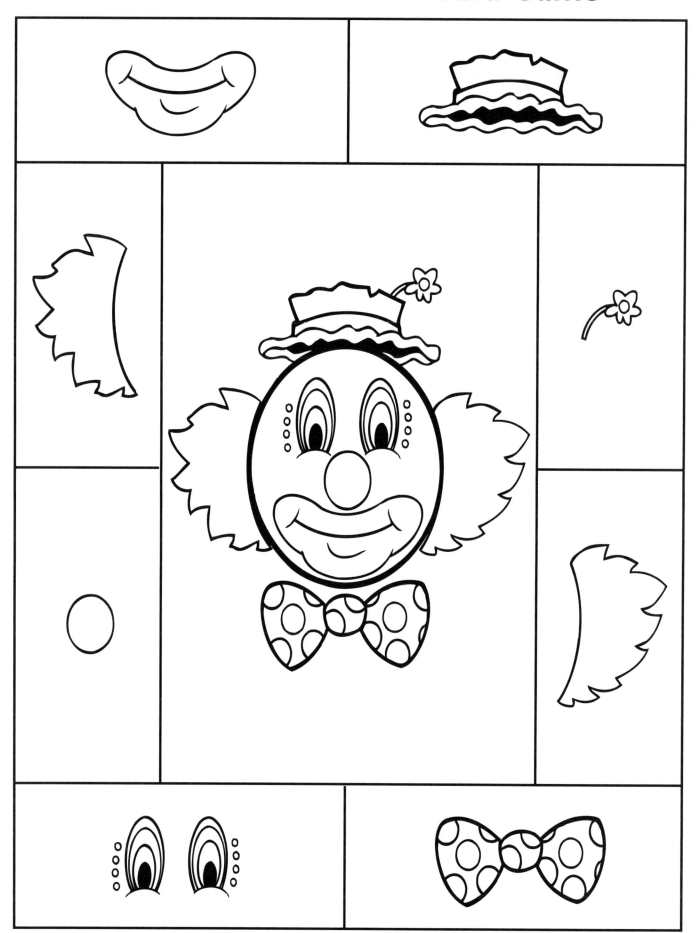

 #BK-272 Year-Round Literature • ©1999 Super Duper® Publications • 1-800-277-8737 • www.superduperinc.com

# Decorate the Clown Student Sheet

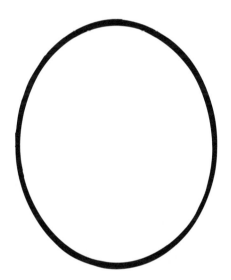

# Circus Matching Game

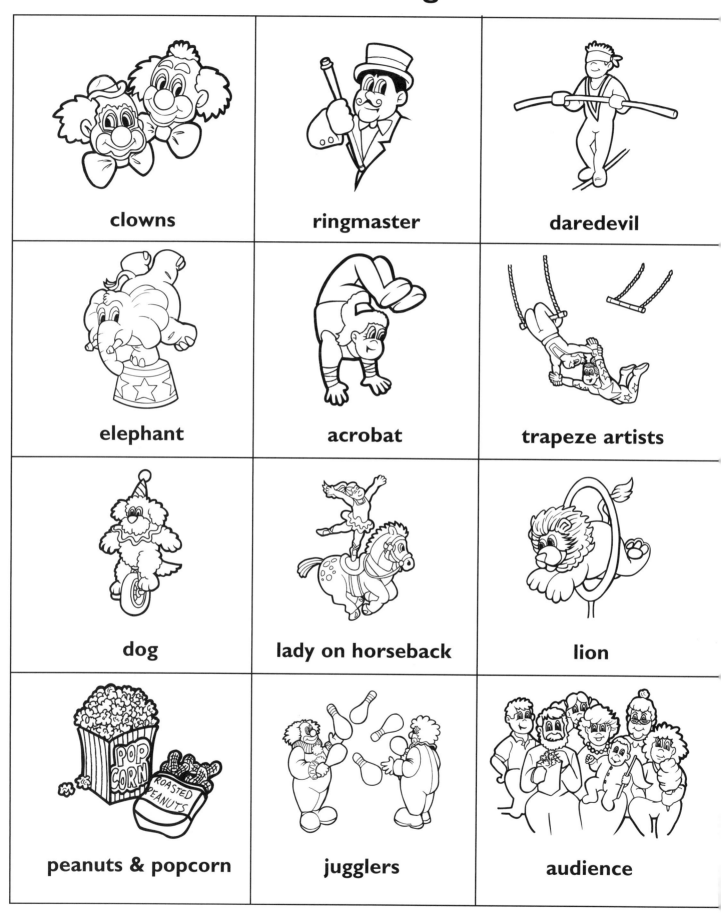

clowns

ringmaster

daredevil

elephant

acrobat

trapeze artists

dog

lady on horseback

lion

peanuts & popcorn

jugglers

audience

#BK-272  Year-Round Literature  •  ©1999 Super Duper® Publications  •  1-800-277-8737  •  www.superduperinc.com

# Ringmaster Game

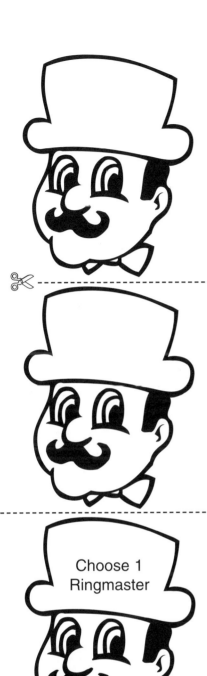

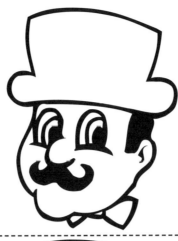

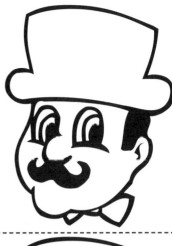

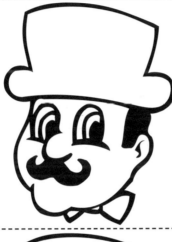

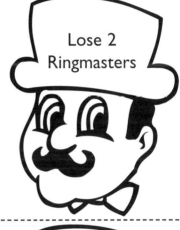
Lose 2 Ringmasters

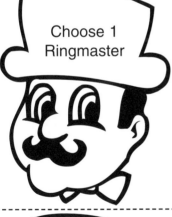
Choose 1 Ringmaster

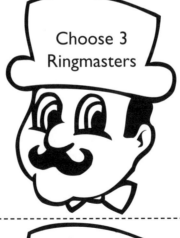
Choose 3 Ringmasters

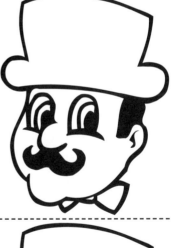

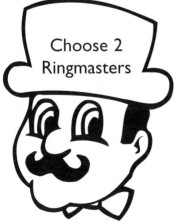
Choose 2 Ringmasters

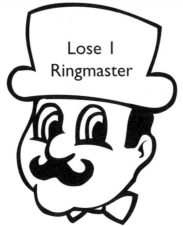
Lose 1 Ringmaster

# Barrier Game

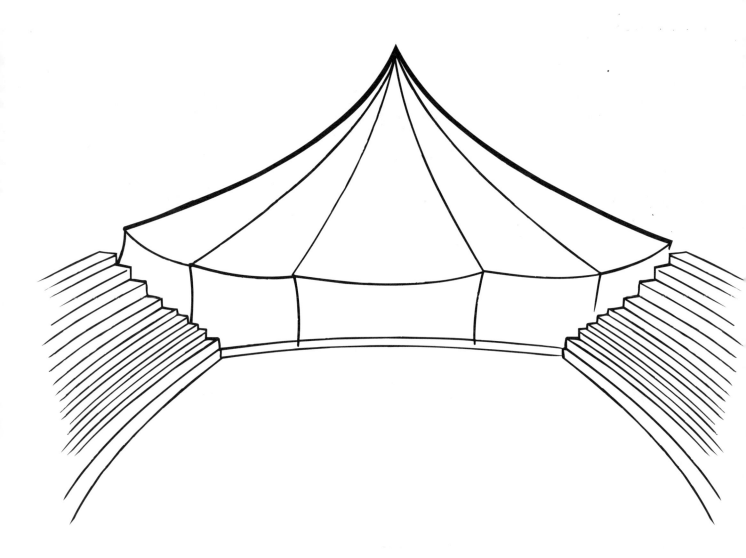

#BK-272  Year-Round Literature  •  ©1999 Super Duper® Publications  •  1-800-277-8737  •  www.superduperinc.com

# Barrier Game

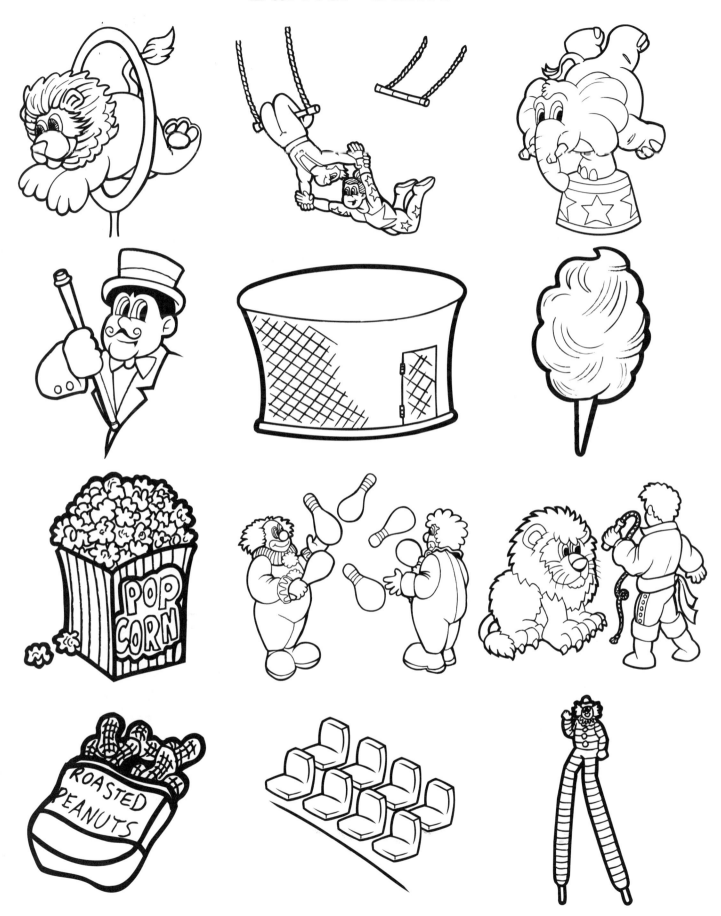

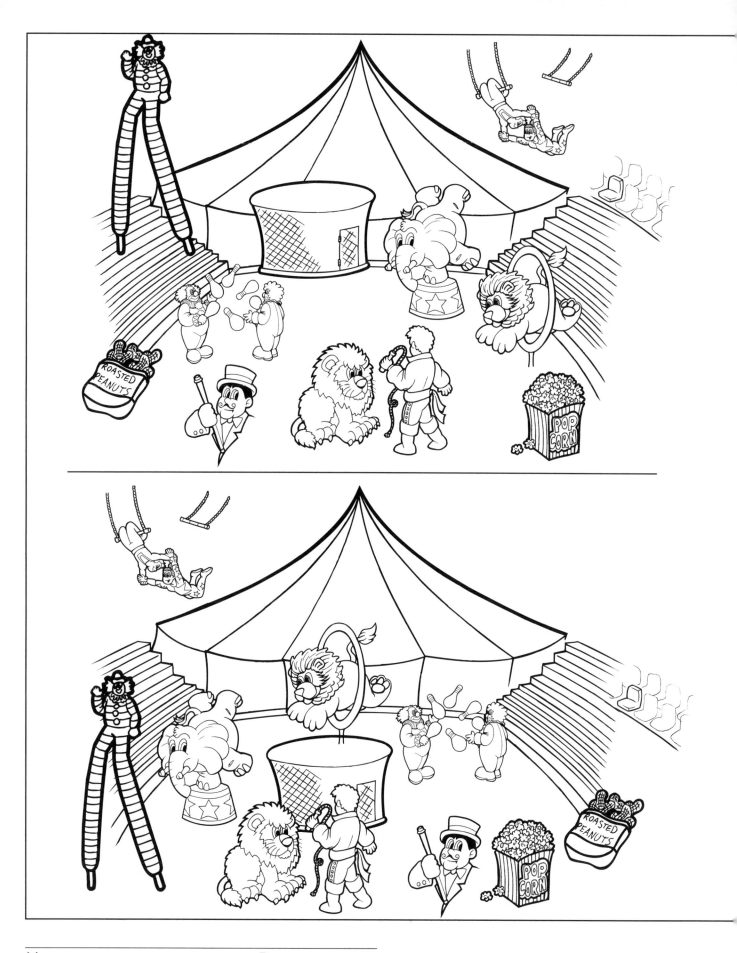

Name _____ Date _____

Speech-Language Pathologist                    Helper's Signature

#BK-272  Year-Round Literature  •  ©1999 Super Duper® Publications  •  1-800-277-8737  •  www.superduperinc.com

# Where's the Circus? Game

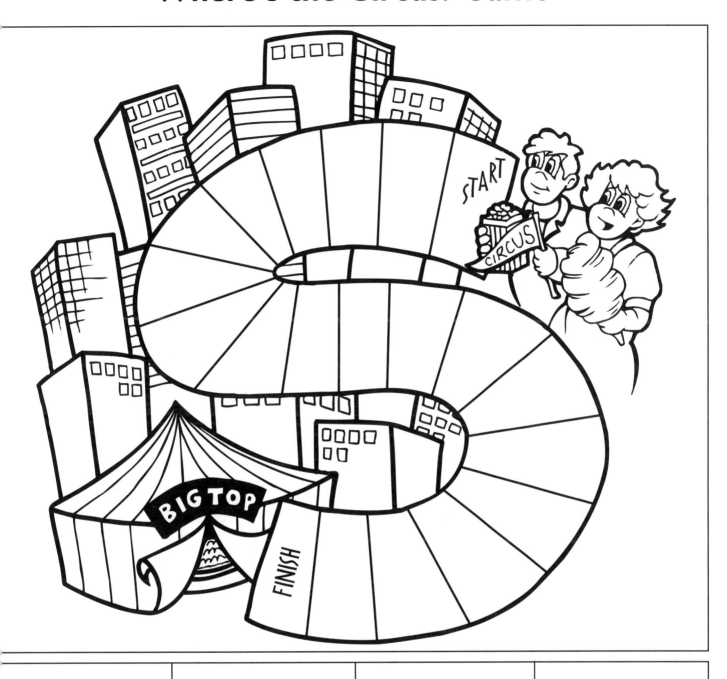

| You have a front row seat. Go forward 3 steps. | You're late for the circus. Go backward 3 steps. | You can't wait to see the performers and the animals. Go forward 2 steps. | Lost your ticket. Go backward 2 steps. |
| --- | --- | --- | --- |
| The circus is starting. Go forward 1 step. | Can't find your seat. Go backward 1 step. | Traffic is heavy. Stay where you are. | You've been chosen to do an act with the clowns. Go forward 1 step. |

# Clowning Around with Good Speech

Write words with _____ in each of the clown's juggling balls. Then, make a sentence with each word out loud using your good speech.

#BK-272  Year-Round Literature  •  ©1999 Super Duper® Publications  •  1-800-277-8737  •  www.superduperinc.com

# It's Circus Time!

Find each circus pictures hidden in the picture below. Then, make a sentence out loud telling about each circus picture. Be sure to use your good speech and language!

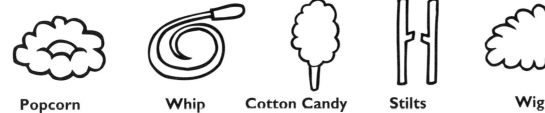

**Popcorn**   **Whip**   **Cotton Candy**   **Stilts**   **Wig**   **Unicycle**

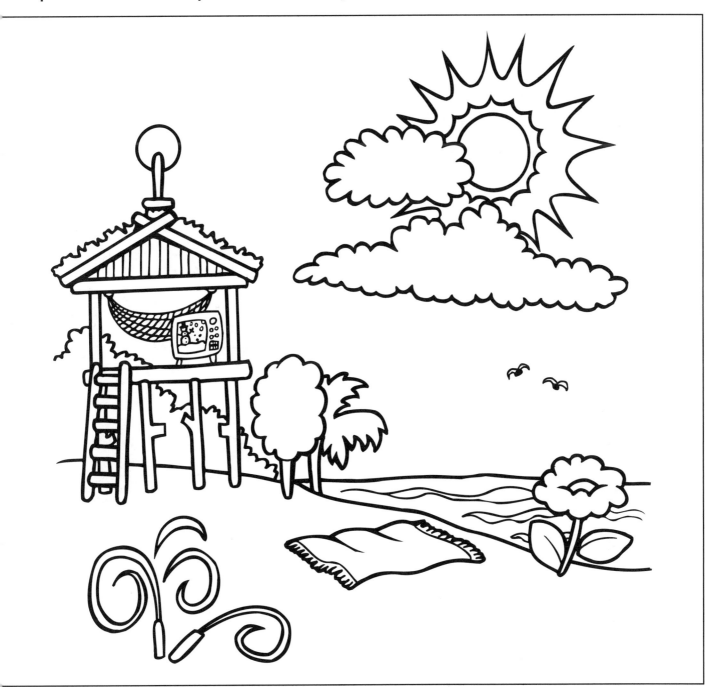

Name _____   Date _____

Speech-Language Pathologist _____   Helper's Signature _____

#BK-272  Year-Round Literature  •  ©1999 Super Duper® Publications  •  1-800-277-8737  •  www.superduperinc.com

# Circus Fun

Tell what is happening in each circus picture below. Which picture do you think shows the most fun? Why? Tell three things that you like about the circus.

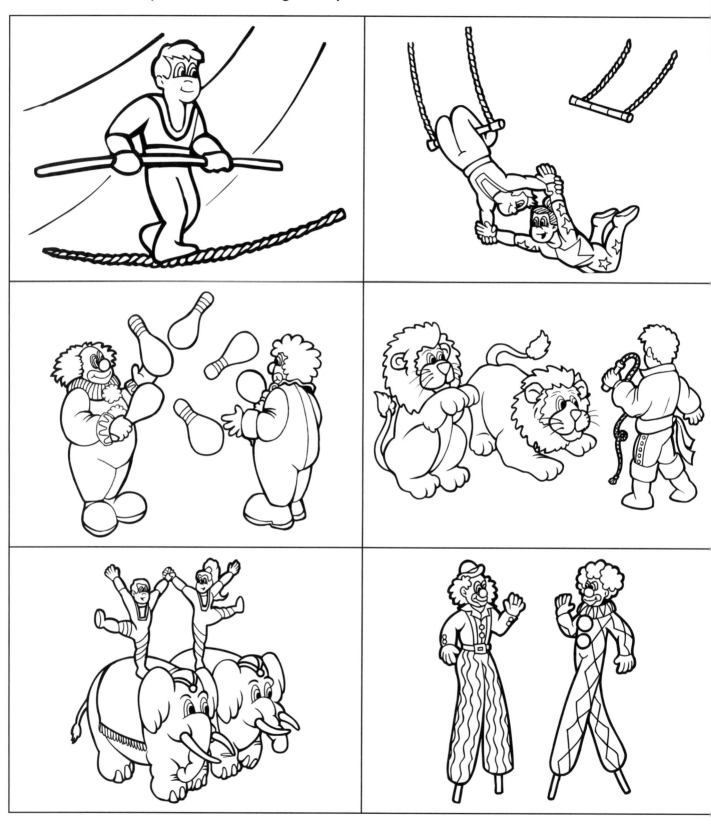

Name _____     Date _____

# Our Bodies

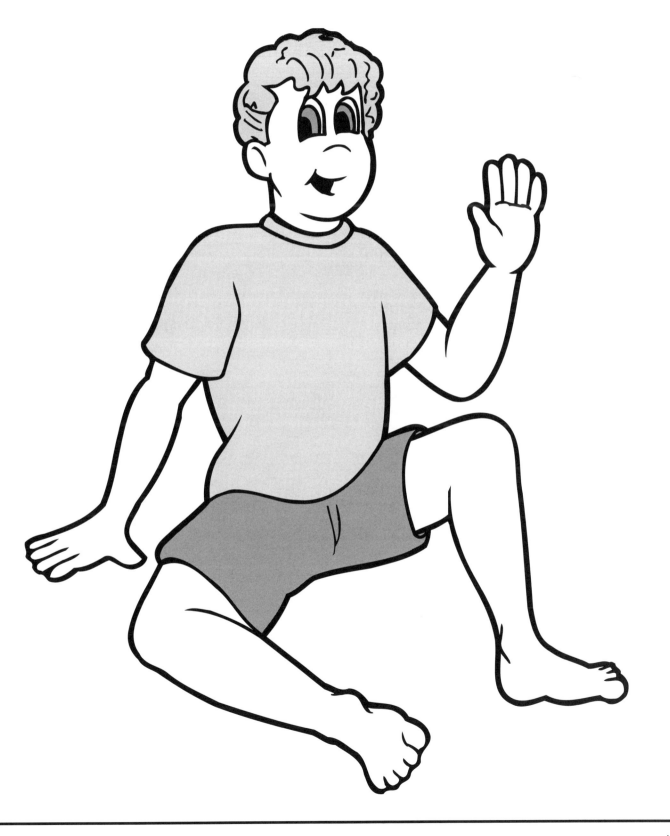

# Our Bodies Articulation & Vocabulary Word Lists

These word lists are a good resource for articulation and/or vocabulary building activities.

## /r/ and /r/ blends

### Initial
right hand
ring
rough
reflex

### Medial
fingernails
forehead
fingerprint
energy
artery
iris
exercise
temperature

### Final
finger
hair
shoulder
hear
shiver
bladder
eye color
whisper
snore
doctor
liver

### Blends
stretch
prickly
scratch
braids
toothbrush
eyebrow
breath
brain
triceps
frown
fruits
grains
cry
freckles
wrist
wrinkles
ambidextrous

ears
heart
nerves
vertebrae
cartilage
nutrition
heartbeat

## /s/ and /s/ blends

### Initial
sign language
see
saliva
senses
sick

### Medial
index finger
sensitive
muscles
tonsils
goose bump
glasses
senses
oxygen
exercise

### Final
ambidextrous
cheeks
fruits
triceps
biceps
iris
voice
pulse
reflex

### Blends
stretch
snap
sticky
scratch
sneeze
stomach
spine
smile
snore

skeleton
smell
sleep
special
skull
swallow
stethoscope
chest
taste
muscles
tonsils
intestines
dentist
whisper
wrist

## /z/

### Medial
dizzy

### Final
hands
fingers
fingernails
wrinkles
knuckles
veins
bones
braids
toes
toenails
shoulders
nose
eyes
ears
eyelashes
eyebrows
freckles
ankles
muscles
tonsils
glasses
lungs
intestines
nerves
organs
vegetables

#BK-272  Year-Round Literature  •  ©1999 Super Duper® Publications  •  1-800-277-8737  •  www.superduperinc.com

# Our Bodies Articulation & Vocabulary Word Lists (Cont.)

## /l/ and /l/ blends

### Initial
left hand
language
leg
liver
lungs

### Medial
swallow
eyelashes
saliva
eye color
cartilage
eyelid
skeleton

### Final
pull
tickle
female
male
smell
muscle
tonsil
feel
skull
smile
cell

### Blends
ankle
pupil
blush
blowing
sleep
shoulder blade
blink
glasses
blood
ankle
reflex
pulse
freckles
prickly
fingernails
cold
healthy
knuckles
elbow
toenails
shoulder

## /k/ and /k/ blends

### Initial
cartilage
cough
kidney
catch
cold

### Medial
eye color
pinky finger
sticky
hiccup

### Final
sick
blink
wink
choke
headache
stomach
back
neck
think
talk

### Blends
skull
cry
skeleton
scratch
skin
exercise
reflex/oxygen
wrinkles
knuckles
tickle
ankle
freckles
doctor

## /g/ and /g/ blends

### Final
hug

### Blends
glasses
grains
organs

fingernail
fingerprint

## /th/ and /th/ blends

### Initial
thermometer
thumb
thigh
think

### Medial
toothbrush
toothpaste
tooth fairy
stethoscope

### Final
smooth
mouth
tooth
teeth
breath
breathe

### Blends
throw
healthy

## /sh/

### Initial
shoulders
shoulder blade
shiver
shout
short hair

### Medial
special
eyelashes

### Final
blush
push

# Our Bodies Articulation & Vocabulary Word Lists (Cont.)

## /ch/

### Initial
chest
cheeks
chew
choke

### Medial
temperature

### Final
catch
stretch
touch
scratch
itch

## /m/ and /m/ blends

### Initial
mouth
muscles
meat
milk
male
move

### Medial
stomach
female

### Blends
smooth
ambidextrous
smell
thumb
palm
goose bump
pump
Adam's apple
smile
temperature

## /p/ and /p/ blends

### Initial
pinky finger
push
pull
ponytail
pump
pupil
pulse

### Final
sleep
snap
hiccup
hip
goose bump
pump
stethoscope

### Blends
prickly
spine
special
fingerprint
Adam's Apple
biceps
triceps
pupil
whisper
temperature

## /b/ and /b/ blends

### Initial
body
biceps
button
bones
back

### Medial
goose bump
heartbeat
ambidextrous

### Blends
shoulder blade
blood
bladder
brain
blush
blink
braids
blowing nose
toothbrush
bruise
vertebrae

vegetables
toothbrush
eyebrows
elbow

## /f/ and /f/ blends

### Initial
fingers
fingernails
feet
face
feel
forehead
food
female

### Final
cough

### Blends
freckles
frown
fruit
soft

## /v/ and /v/ blends

### Initial
veins
vertebrae

### Medial
shiver
saliva
liver

### Final
move

### Blends
nerves

#BK-272 Year-Round Literature • ©1999 Super Duper® Publications • 1-800-277-8737 • www.superduperinc.com

# Vocabulary Pictures

Instructions: _____

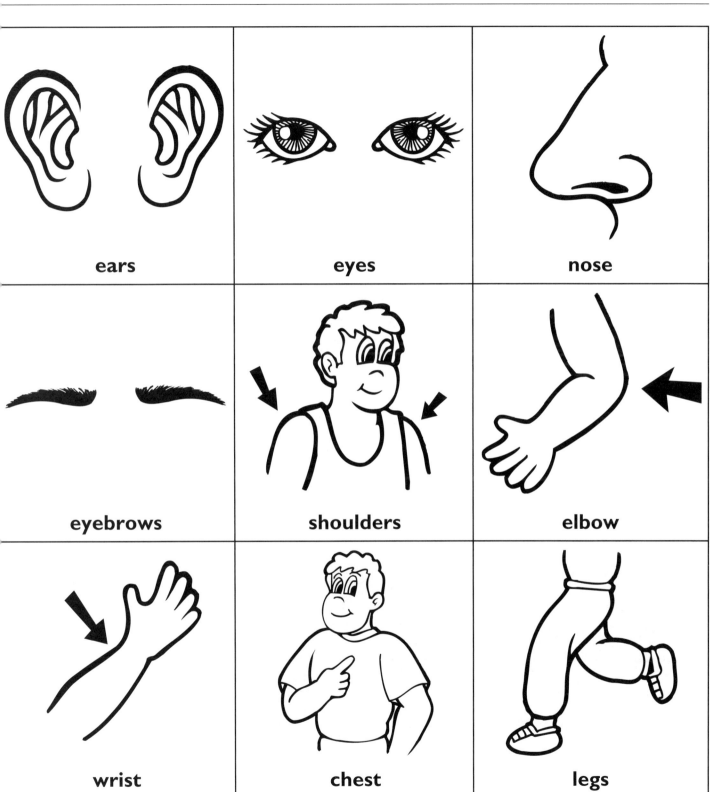

| | | |
|---|---|---|
| **ears** | **eyes** | **nose** |
| **eyebrows** | **shoulders** | **elbow** |
| **wrist** | **chest** | **legs** |

Name _____  Date _____

# Vocabulary Pictures

**Instructions:** _____

_____

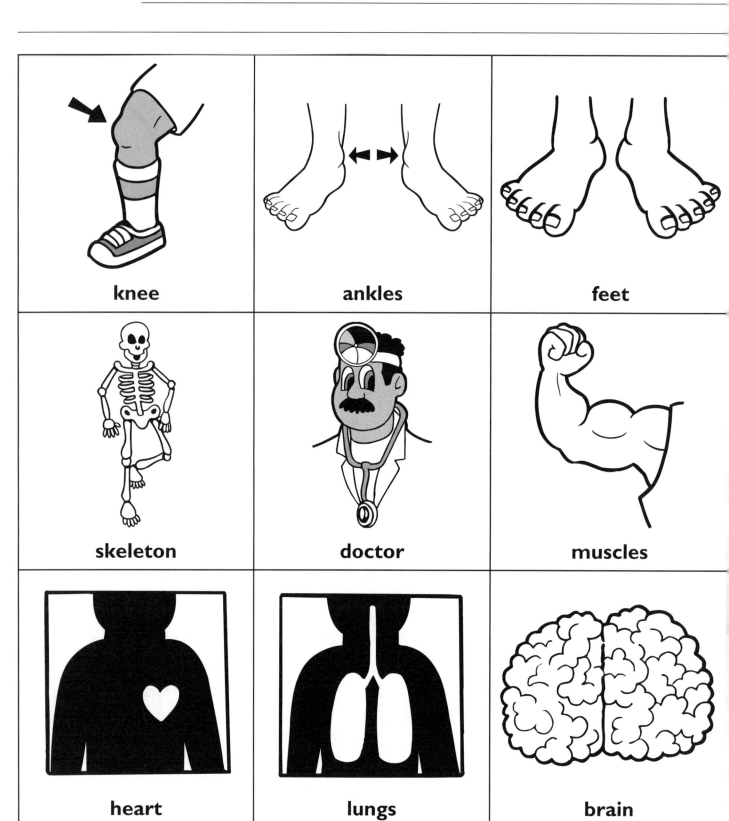

| | | |
|---|---|---|
| **knee** | **ankles** | **feet** |
| **skeleton** | **doctor** | **muscles** |
| **heart** | **lungs** | **brain** |

Name _____ Date _____

_____

# Vocabulary Pictures

Instructions: _____

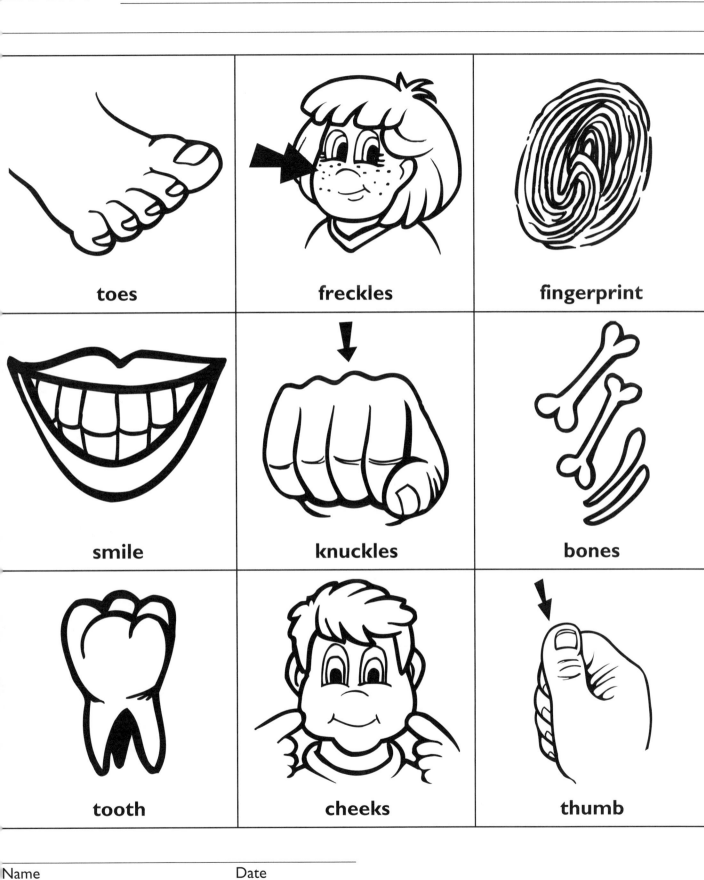

| | | |
|---|---|---|
| toes | freckles | fingerprint |
| smile | knuckles | bones |
| tooth | cheeks | thumb |

Name _____  Date _____

# Story Pattern

**Name:**

Name                    Date

Speech-Language Pathologist          Helper's Signature

# *From Head to Toe*
## by Eric Carle

This book discusses a variety of animals moving different body parts and then asks the reader to move his body parts as well. The parts addressed in the book include: the head, neck, shoulders, arms, hands, chest, back, hips, knees, legs, feet, and toes. This book is quite appropriate for younger elementary students.

**Language Expansion:** The following questions can be used to address students' recall of this book or to expand upon concepts addressed in this book.

## Definition
1. What is your head?
2. What is your neck?
3. What are your hands?
4. What is your chest?
5. What is your foot?

## Function
1. What can you do with your head?
2. What are arms used for?
3. What are hands used for?
4. What are knees used for?
5. What are legs used for?

## Category
1. Name three parts of your body.
2. Name three parts of your face.
3. Name three of the finger names.
4. Name three things you can do with your hands.
5. Name three things you can do with your feet.

## Description
1. Tell me three things about your head.
2. Tell me three things about your shoulders.
3. Tell me three things about your hands
4. Tell me three things about your back.
5. Tell me three things about your body.

## Vocabulary
Make a sentence using the following words.
1. neck
2. shoulders
3. chest
4. back
5. hips

## Rhyming
Name a rhyming word for each word below.
1. head
2. hand
3. feet
4. back
5. hip

## Sequencing
As your students sequence the events in this story, use this list as a guide.
1. The book talks about your head.
2. The book talks about your shoulders.
3. The book talks about your hands.
4. The book talks about your hips.
5. The book talks about your toes.

# My Hands
## by Aliki

This is a book that describes the many ways that we can use our hands. Some examples include touching objects, holding things, and playing with toys. The book also introduces concepts and vocabulary such as left hand and right hand, the names of the fingers, and much more.

**Language Expansion:** The following questions can be used to address students' recall of this book or to expand upon concepts addressed in this book.

## Definition
1. What are hands?
2. What are fingers?
3. What is the palm of your hand?
4. What is a bone?
5. What is a knuckle?

## Function
1. What is a hand used for?
2. What are fingers used for?
3. What is a ring finger used for?
4. What is a fingernail for?
5. What is a thumb used for?

## Category
1. Name three things you can do with your hands.
2. Name three parts of your hands.
3. Name three of the finger names.
4. Name three things you can do with your thumbs.
5. Name three things about your palms.

## Description
1. Tell me three things about your hands.
2. Tell me three things about your fingers.
3. Tell me three things about your fingernails.
4. Tell me three things about your thumbs.
5. Tell me three things about your palms.

## Vocabulary
Make a sentence using the following words.
1. ambidextrous
2. veins
3. music
4. deaf/sign language
5. manners

## Rhyming
Name a rhyming word for each word below.
1. bone
2. vein
3. ring
4. play
5. hold

## Sequencing
As your students sequence the events in this story, use this list as a guide.
1. The book talks about your hands playing peek-a-boo.
2. The book tells the names of your five fingers.
3. The book talks about your fingers having fingernails.
4. The book talks about the palms of your hands.
5. The book talks about how every hand is different and how your hands help you do many things.

#BK-272 Year-Round Literature • ©1999 Super Duper® Publications • 1-800-277-8737 • www.superduperinc.com

# Here Are My Hands
## by Bill Martin, Jr. and John Archambault

This book about the body is for younger children. It addresses the purposes of body parts, including: hands, feet, head, nose, eyes, ears, knees, cheeks, teeth, elbows, and skin.

**Language Expansion:** The following questions can be used to address students' recall of this book or to expand upon concepts addressed in this book.

## Definition
1. What are hands?
2. What are feet?
3. What is a nose?
4. What are eyes?
5. What are ears?

## Function
1. What are hands used for?
2. What is a nose used for?
3. What are eyes used for?
4. What are ears used for?
5. What are teeth used for?

## Category
1. Name three things you can do with your hands.
2. Name three things you can do with your feet.
3. Name three things you can see with your eyes.
4. Name three things you can hear with your ears.
5. Name three things you can smell with your nose.

## Description
1. Tell me three things about your hands.
2. Tell me three things about your feet.
3. Tell me three things about your head.
4. Tell me three things about your eyes.
5. Tell me three things about your teeth.

## Vocabulary
Make a sentence using the following words.
1. knees
2. neck
3. cheeks
4. elbow
5. skin

## Rhyming
Name a rhyming word for each word below.
1. nose
2. ear
3. skin
4. cheek
5. see

## Sequencing
As your students sequence the events in this story, use this list as a guide.

1. The book talks about how your hands are for catching and throwing.
2. The book talks about how your feet are for stopping and going.
3. The book talks about how your head is for thinking and knowing.
4. The book talks about how your nose is for smelling and blowing.
5. The book talks about how your eyes are for seeing and crying.
6. The book talks about how your ears are for washing and drying.
7. The book talks about how your knees are for falling down.
8. The book talks about how your neck is for turning around.
9. The book talks about how your cheeks are for kissing and blushing.
10. The book talks about how your teeth are for chewing and brushing.
11. The book talks about how your skin bundles you in.

# Our Bodies Articulation and Language Games
(The following games can be used with the articulation and vocabulary word list or the literature language questions.)

## Senses Category Game

Divide a piece of poster board into five sections or use five pieces of paper. Label each piece of paper with one of the five senses —smell, touch, sight, hearing and taste. This will be your game board. Copy, color, cut out, and laminate the senses game cards (pages 137 and 138). Turn the cards over and lay them flat on the table. After each student makes a sentence with a body word containing his/her sound or answers a body language question, the student may then choose a card from the pile. Have the student place the card in a category section and tell why he/she chose to put the card in that particular category section of the game board. The object of the game is for the team to have all the game cards placed in the correct category sections of the game board by the end of class.

### Language Extension

Ask the students to brainstorm other pictures that might belong in each section. Talk about parts of the body that are used for each sense. Discuss how many things are perceived by several senses.

## Parts of the Body Game

Make one copy of the Parts of the Body (page 139) for each student. Color, cut out, and laminate each body part. Put all of the cards in a bucket or bowl. After a student makes a sentence with a body word containing his/her sound or answers a body language question, the student may draw a card from the bucket or bowl. The object of the game is for each student to get all the body parts by the end of the session.

### Language Extension

After collecting all of the parts of the body, have each student describe each part and tell what each part is used for. Talk about unusual things you can do with each part.

### Team Approach

In order to win the game, each team member must collect all of the parts of a body by the end of class.

## Parts of a Face Game

Photocopy, color, and laminate the following game board (page 140). Then, photocopy the student sheet (page 141) for each student. (You can photocopy front and back to paper and use the back side with the next therapy group.) Make a game die using a penny. Put a piece of masking tape on both sides and write a "2" on one side and a "3" on the other side with permanent ink.

Discuss the different parts of the face on the game board and tell the class that the goal is for each student to get each part to complete the face on the student sheet. Give each child a student sheet and a pencil. After a student makes a sentence with a body word containing his/her sound or answers a body language question, the student may flip the penny die, move the allotted number of spaces and draw the part of the face on the student sheet.

### Language Extension

After completing the face, ask the student to name the parts of the face and tell the purpose of each part.

## Hand Game

Make copies of the hand pattern (page 142) on construction paper. Laminate the hands. Place hands number side down on the table. After a student makes a sentence with a body word containing his/her sound or answers a body language question, the student may draw a hand. The number on the back is the number of points the student receives on the score sheet for the turn. The student with the most points wins.

### Team Approach

In order to win the game, the team must earn a number of points. For example, the team must have 30 points by the end of class to win.

## Body Matching Game

Make two copies of the body matching game (page 143). Color the parts of the body, cut them out, and laminate them. Lay the cards facedown and allow each student to turn over two cards. If the cards don't match, the student must choose one of the cards to name and describe using good speech and language and then put both cards facedown. If the cards match, the student must tell about the body part by naming and describing it using good speech and language. Then, the student may keep the matching pair. Continue taking turns until all of the body parts have been matched. The student with the most matches is the winner.

### Team Approach

In order to win the game, the team must be able to match all of the body parts by the end of the therapy session.

 #BK-272 Year-Round Literature • ©1999 Super Duper® Publications • 1-800-277-8737 • www.superduperinc.com

# Senses Category Game

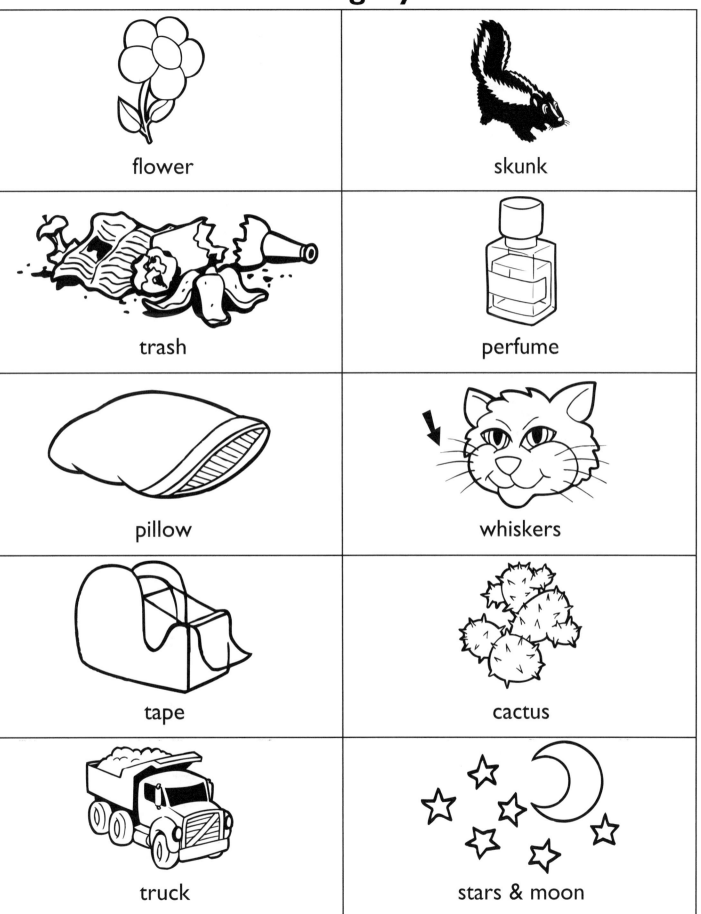

| flower | skunk |
| --- | --- |
| trash | perfume |
| pillow | whiskers |
| tape | cactus |
| truck | stars & moon |

# Senses Category Game

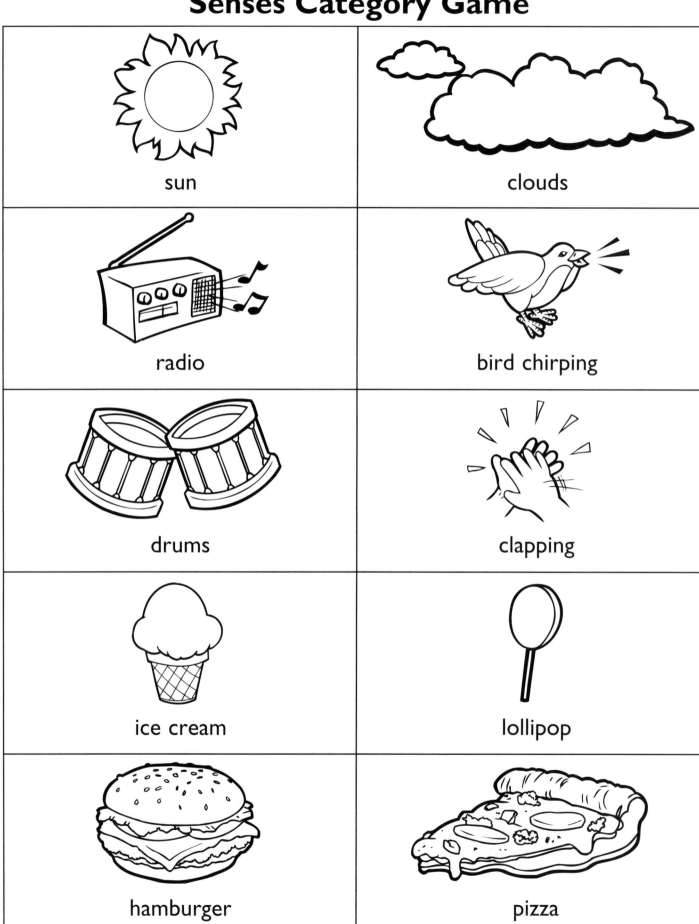

| | |
|---|---|
| sun | clouds |
| radio | bird chirping |
| drums | clapping |
| ice cream | lollipop |
| hamburger | pizza |

#BK-272  Year-Round Literature  •  ©1999 Super Duper® Publications  •  1-800-277-8737  •  www.superduperinc.com

# Parts of the Body Game

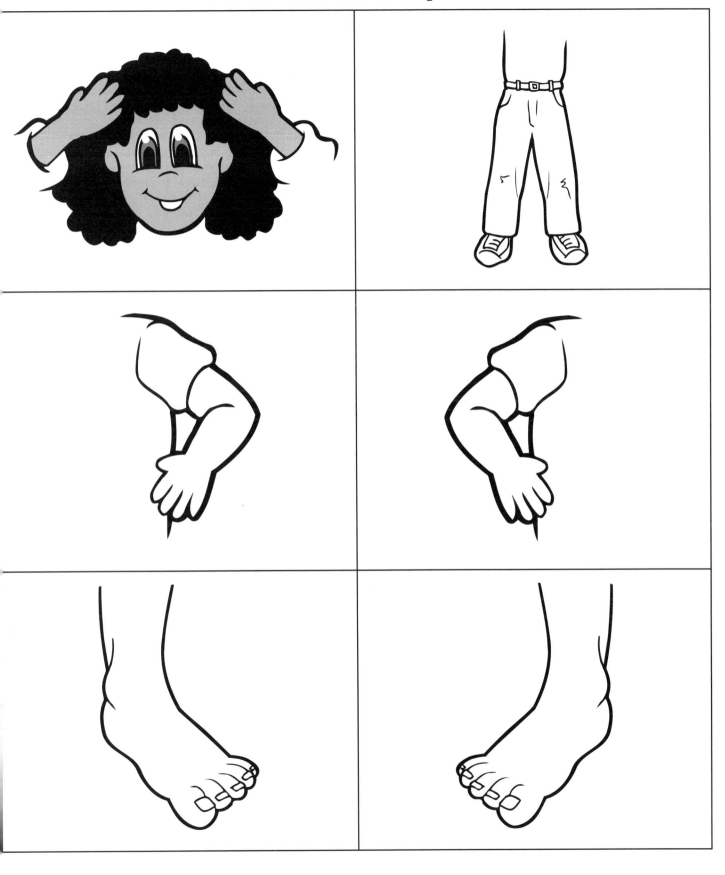

Name _____    Date _____

Speech-Language Pathologist    Helper's Signature

#BK-272  Year-Round Literature  •  ©1999 Super Duper® Publications  •  1-800-277-8737  •  www.superduperinc.com    139

# Parts of a Face Board Game

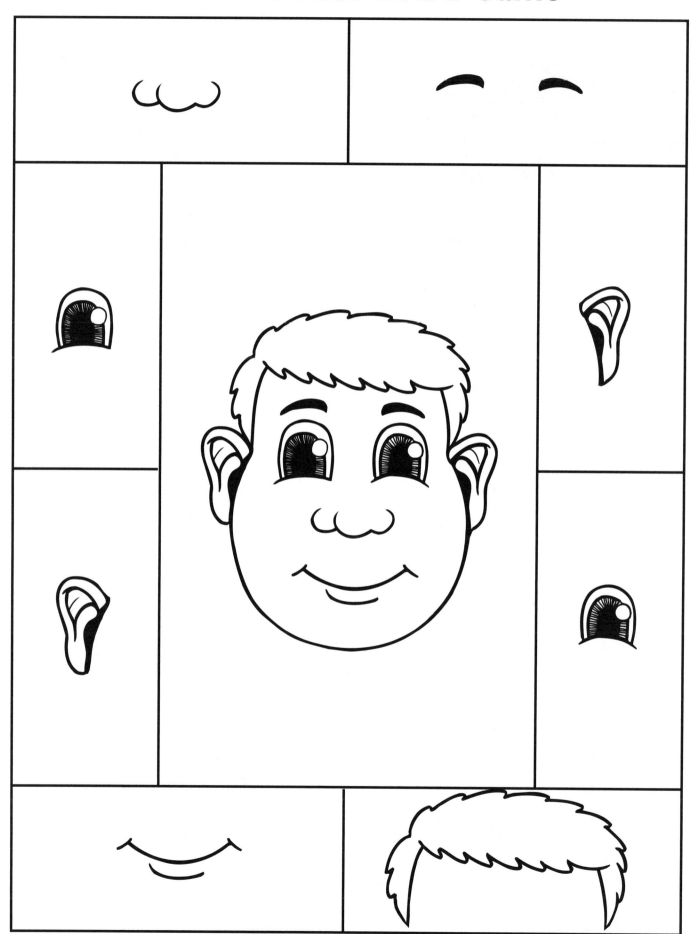

#BK-272  Year-Round Literature  •  ©1999 Super Duper® Publications  •  1-800-277-8737  •  www.superduperinc.com

# Parts of a Face Student Sheet

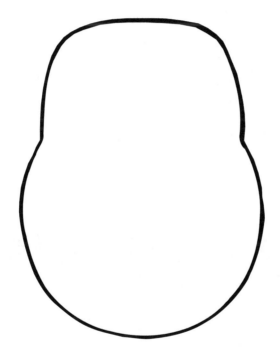

# Hands Game

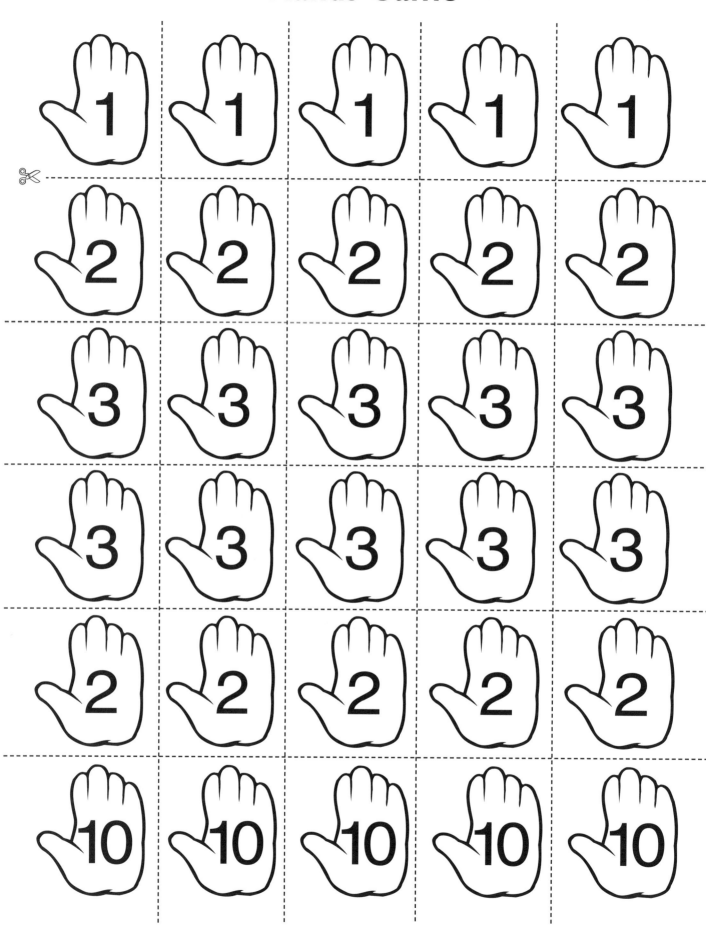

#BK-272   Year-Round Literature   •   ©1999 Super Duper® Publications   •   1-800-277-8737   •   www.superduperinc.com

# Body Matching Game

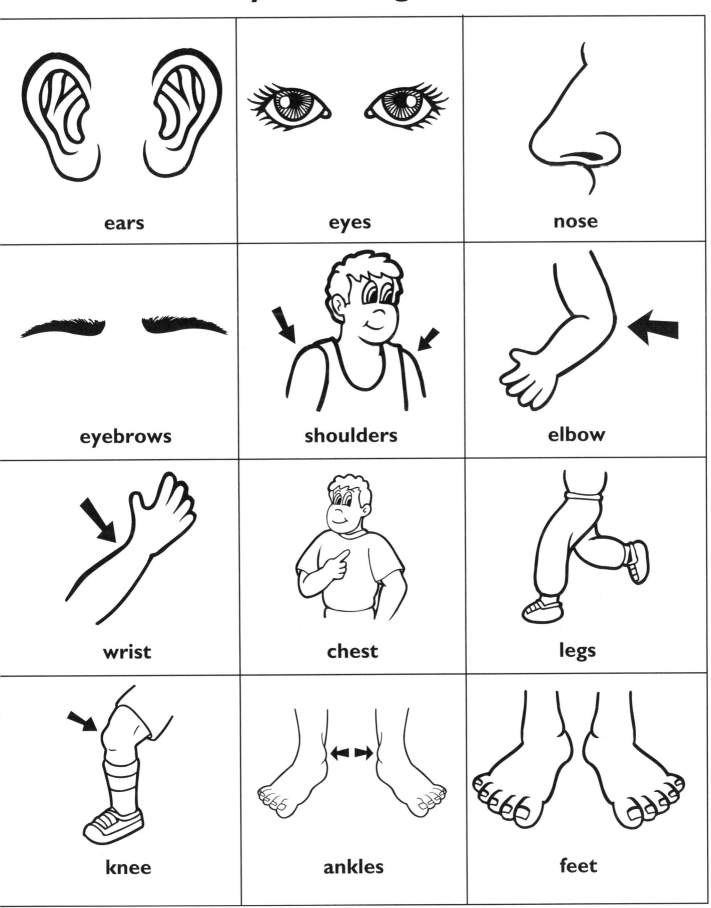

ears

eyes

nose

eyebrows

shoulders

elbow

wrist

chest

legs

knee

ankles

feet

# A Handful of Good Speech

Write words with _____ in each hand. Then, make a sentence with each word out loud using your good speech.

Name _____

Date _____

Speech-Language Pathologist

Helper's Signature

# Parts of the Body

Can you name each part of the body? Cut out the words below and put them in the correct place.

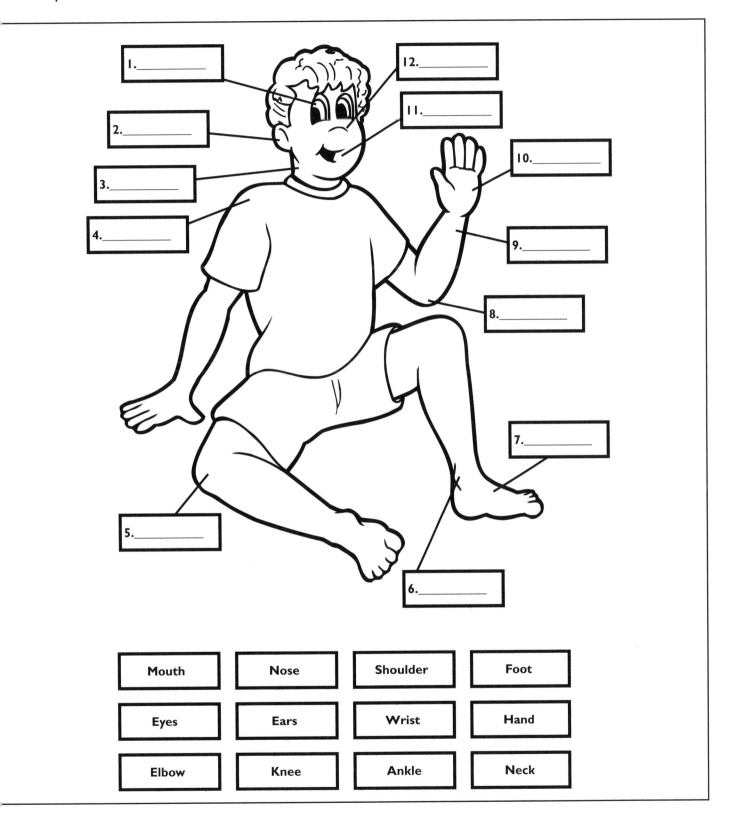

1. _____
2. _____
3. _____
4. _____
5. _____
6. _____
7. _____
8. _____
9. _____
10. _____
11. _____
12. _____

| Mouth | Nose | Shoulder | Foot |
| Eyes | Ears | Wrist | Hand |
| Elbow | Knee | Ankle | Neck |

Name _____    Date _____

Speech-Language Pathologist                Helper's Signature

# Our Amazing Bodies

Tell what is happening in each picture below. What parts of the body are being used?
What senses are being used in each picture? Use your good speech.

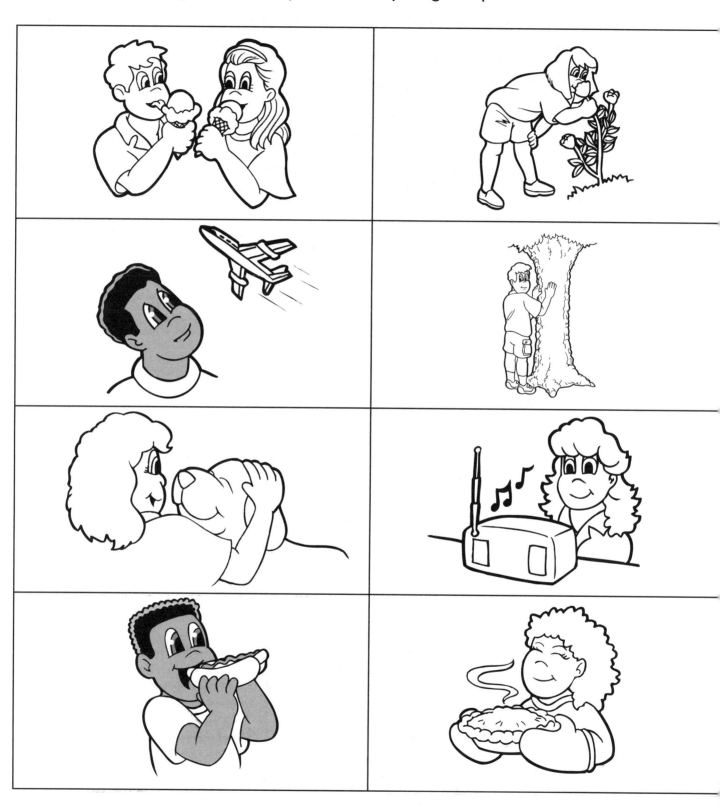

Name _____ Date _____

Speech-Language Pathologist _____ Helper's Signature _____

#BK-272  Year-Round Literature  •  ©1999 Super Duper® Publications  •  1-800-277-8737  •  www.superduperinc.com

# Farm

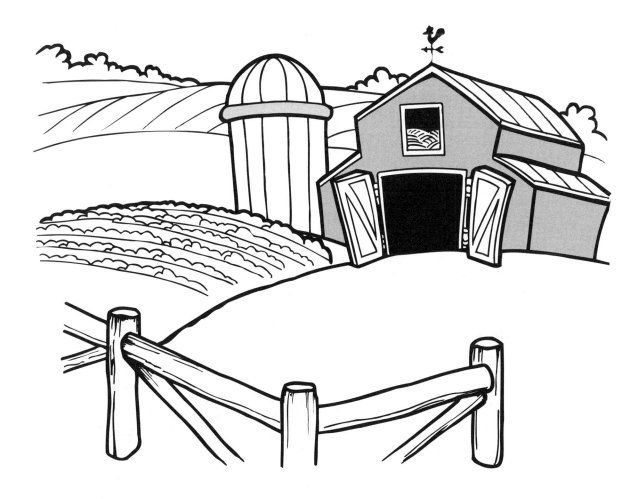

# Farm Articulation & Vocabulary Word Lists

These word lists are a good resource for articulation and/or vocabulary building activities.

## /r/ and /r/ blends

### Initial
rope
rooster
rake

### Medial
overalls
carrot
turkey
dairy
harvest
veterinarian
wheelbarrow

### Final
hair
pasture
udder
fur
feather
store

### Blends
bark
crops
grass
stream
frog
drink
grow
tractor
grain
graze
straw
trough
corn
farm
barn
dirt
scarecrow
shirt
horse
pitchfork
horns
corn mush

## /s/ and /s/ blends

### Initial
silo
sow
seeds
socks
sell

### Final
fence
horse
house
socks
boots
goose

### Blends
harvest
slop
stool
scarecrow
sweater
sleeves
stable
store
straw
pig sty
haystack
stream
rooster
pasture

## /z/

### Initial
zucchini

### Medial
dozen

### Final
hooves
chickens
seeds
cheese
animals
peas
gloves
sleeves
graze

## and /l/ blends

### Initial
lettuce
lamb
lay

### Medial
duckling
hay loft
lily pad
silo
wheelbarrow

### Final
bale
tail
tad pole
sell
animal
apple
foal
wool
stool

### Blends
slop
play
plow
fly
clothespin
clothes line
clothes
piglet
stable

## /k/ and /k/ blends

### Initial
corn
cat
kitten
kid
calf
coop
cock-a-doodle-doo
cow

### Medial
corn on the cob
chicken

turkey
cock-a-doodle-doo

### Final
duck
chick
haystack
pick
drink
oink
bark

### Blends
quack
duckling
milk
socks

## /g/

### Initial
goat
gate
goose

### Medial
pig pen
wagon

### Final
pig
dog
hog
log
egg
frog

## /th/

### Initial
thermometer
thimble
thorn
thistle

### Medial
feather
weather vane
clothing
bathtub
bathroom

#BK-272  Year-Round Literature  •  ©1999 Super Duper® Publications  •  1-800-277-8737  •  www.superduperinc.com

# Farm Articulation & Vocabulary Word Lists (Cont.)

## /th/ and /th/ blends
### Final
mouth
teeth

## /sh/
### Initial
short-sleeved
shirt
shovel
sheep
shoes

### Medial
bushel
fishing
wishbone
horseshoe

### Final
fish
corn mush
squash

## /ch/
### Initial
chickens
chick
chop
cheese
chin
churn
chimney
chicken coop

### Medial
pitcher
orchard
kitchen
hatchet
rocking chair

### Final
bench

## /m/ and /m/ blends
### Initial
milk
man

meow
moo
meat
mouse

### Medial
hammer
tomato

### Final
broom

### Blends
pumpkin
comb
worm

## /p/ and /p/ blends
### Initial
pie
pig
piglet
pen
pumpkin
pasture
pick
pond

### Medial
puppy

### Final
coop
sheep
slop

### Blends
plow
plant
pumpkin

## /b/ and /b/ blends
### Initial
bed
bird
barn
boots
bark
bale
### Medial

baby animals
### Final
corn on the cob

### Blends
stable

## /f/
### Initial
feather
fence
food
fur
foal
feed
field

### Medial
pitchfork

### Final
calf
hoof
roof
trough

## /v/ and /v/ blends
### Initial
veterinarian

### Medial
weather vane
hooves
harvest

### Final
glove
sleeve
stove

### Blends
calves
hooves
shovel

#BK-272 Year-Round Literature • ©1999 Super Duper® Publications • 1-800-277-8737 • www.superduperinc.com   149

# Vocabulary Pictures

**Instructions:** _____

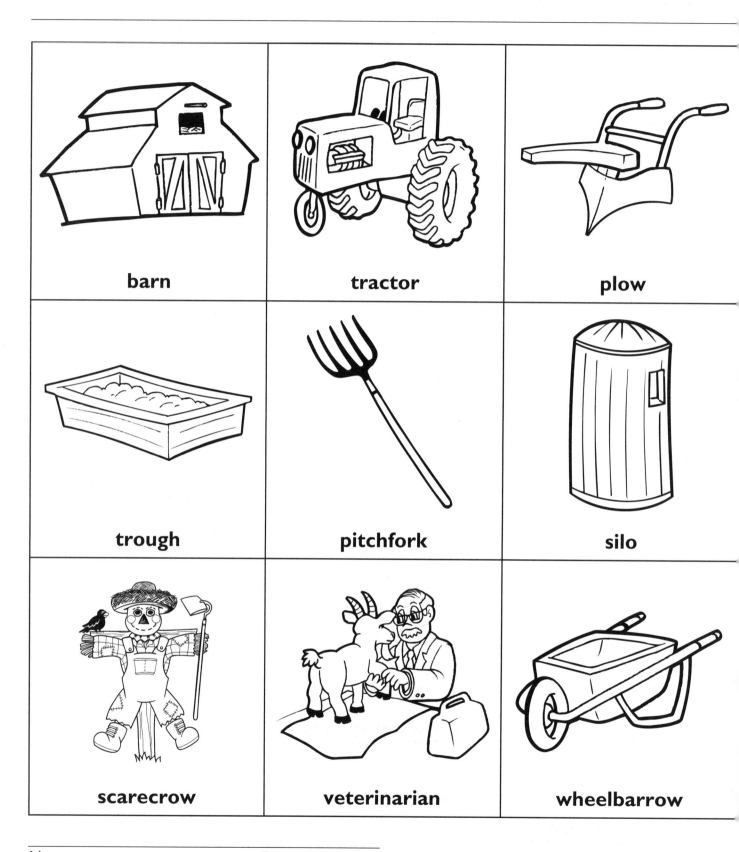

| | | |
|---|---|---|
| barn | tractor | plow |
| trough | pitchfork | silo |
| scarecrow | veterinarian | wheelbarrow |

Name _____    Date _____

Speech-Language Pathologist                    Helper's Signature

#BK-272  Year-Round Literature  • ©1999 Super Duper® Publications • 1-800-277-8737 • www.superduperinc.com

# Vocabulary Pictures

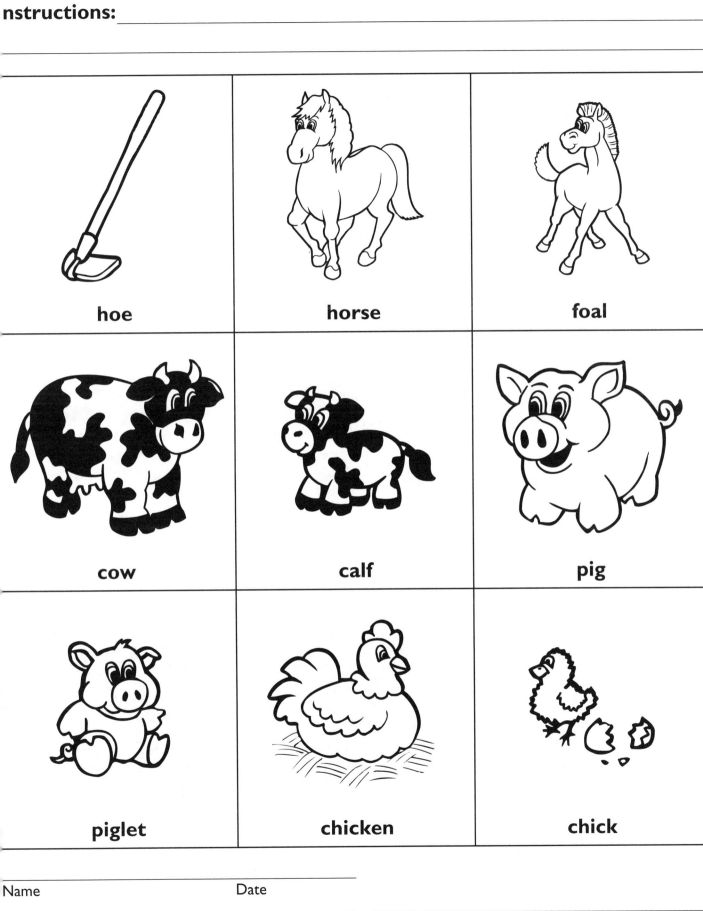

| | | |
|---|---|---|
| hoe | horse | foal |
| cow | calf | pig |
| piglet | chicken | chick |

Name_____ Date_____

Speech-Language Pathologist                    Helper's Signature

# Vocabulary Pictures

**Instructions:** _____

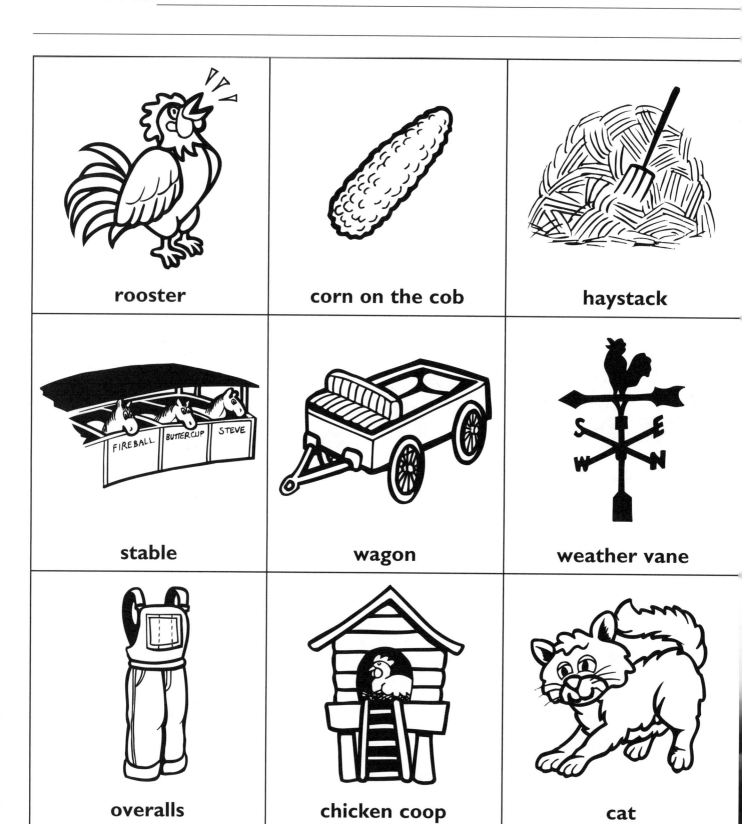

| | | |
|---|---|---|
| rooster | corn on the cob | haystack |
| stable | wagon | weather vane |
| overalls | chicken coop | cat |

Name _____

Date _____

# Story Pattern

**Name:** _____

_____

_____

_____

_____

_____

_____

_____

_____

_____

Name _____    Date _____

Speech-Language Pathologist _____    Helper's Signature _____

# The Day Jimmy's Boa Ate the Wash
## by Trinka Noble and illustrated by Steven Kellogg

Jimmy's class from school takes a field trip to the farm.  The book is quite humorous and has wonderful illustrations that catch any child's attention.

**Language Expansion:**  The following questions can be used to address students' recall of this book or to expand upon concepts addressed in this book.

## Definition
1. What is a farm?
2. What is a barn?
3. What is a haystack?
4. What is a tractor?
5. What is a farmer?

## Function
1. How is a farm used?
2. How is hay used on a farm?
3. What is a tractor used for?
4. What is a hen house used for?
5. What is an egg used for?

## Category
1. Name three class trips you have taken.
2. Name three kinds of farm animals.
3. Name three things that a farmer does.
4. Name three things that a farmer wears.
5. Name three things that you can do with eggs.

## Description
1. Tell me three things about a farm.
2. Tell me three things about a tractor.
3. Tell me three things about a farmer.
4. Tell me three things about a barn.
5. Tell me three things about a pig.

## Vocabulary
Make a sentence using the following words.
1. farm
2. trip
3. haystack
4. boa constrictor
5. tractor

## Rhyming
Name a rhyming word for each word below.
1. farm
2. hay
3. hen
4. pig
5. trip

## Sequencing
As your students sequence the events in this story, use this list as a guide.

1. A little girl's class takes a trip to the farm.
2. A farmer runs into a haystack, which fell on the cow.
3. The pigs eat the kids' lunches on the school bus.
4. The kids throw corn and eggs at each other.
5. Jimmy's boa constrictor escapes from his bag, goes to the hen house, and scares all of the chickens away.
6. A chicken lays an egg on Jenny's head, which starts the egg fight.
7. The boa constrictor goes to the clothesline and begins eating the clothes, which made the farmer's wife scream.
8. The class leaves without the boa constrictor, but one of the pigs doesn't get off the bus so now Jimmy has a pet pig.

#BK-272  Year-Round Literature  •  ©1999 Super Duper® Publications  •  1-800-277-8737  •  www.superduperinc.com

# The Big Red Barn
## by Margaret Brown

This book is about the animals that live in the barn. The happenings around the barn take readers through the cycle of the day at the barn. Activities from sun-up to sun-down are described and illustrated.

**Language Expansion:** The following questions can be used to address students' recall of this book or to expand upon concepts addressed in this book.

## Definition
1. What is a barn?
2. What is a field?
3. What is a weather vane?
4. What is hay?
5. What is a scarecrow?

## Function
1. What is a barn used for?
2. What is a field used for?
3. What is a weather vane used for?
4. What is hay used for?
5. What is a scarecrow used for?

## Category
1. Name three kinds of farm animals.
2. Name three farm and animal noises.
3. Name three things a scarecrow wears.
4. Name three things that grow on a farm.
5. Name three things that you can do with eggs.

## Description
1. Tell me three things about a farm.
2. Tell me three things about a weather vane.
3. Tell me three things about a chicken.
4. Tell me three things about a scarecrow.
5. Tell me three things about a day on the farm.

## Vocabulary
Make a sentence using the following words.
1. barn
2. field
3. weather vane
4. hay
5. scarecrow

## Rhyming
Name a rhyming word for each word below.
1. sun
2. crow
3. day
4. barn
5. red

## Sequencing
As your students sequence the events in this story, use this list as a guide.
1. On the farm, there is a pink pig, a big horse, and a little horse.
2. On the farm, there is a weather vane and a big pile of hay.
3. On the farm, there are sheep, donkeys, geese, and goats.
4. On the farm, there is an old scarecrow in a field of corn.
5. On the farm, there is a rooster, pigeon, and a hen.
6. On the farm, there is a brown cow, black cat, and a big, red dog.

# Barn Dance

## by Bill Martin, Jr. and John Archambault

In an old farmhouse, a boy is about to go to bed when he hears the calling of an owl. He hops out of bed and follows the sound to the barn where the animals are having a barn dance. The book has wonderful illustrations and is written in rhyme.

**Language Expansion:** The following questions can be used to address students' recall of this book or to expand upon concepts addressed in this book.

## Definition
1. What is a farm?
2. What is a barn?
3. What is a farmer?
4. What is music?
5. What is a scarecrow?

## Function
1. What is a farm used for?
2. What is a bed used for?
3. What is a scarecrow used for?
4. What is a fiddle used for?
5. What is a barn used for?

## Category
1. Name three farm animals.
2. Name three things a farmer does.
3. Name three things that the animals did at the dance.
4. Name three instruments.
5. Name three things that the scarecrow was wearing.

## Description
1. Tell me three things about a farm.
2. Tell me three things about a scarecrow.
3. Tell me three things about a barn.
4. Tell me three things about a cow.
5. Tell me three things about a fiddle.

## Vocabulary
Make a sentence using the following words.
1. farm
2. scarecrow
3. fiddle
4. hoe-down
5. barn dance

## Rhyming
Name a rhyming word for each word below
1. fiddle
2. bed
3. dance
4. cow
5. owl

## Sequencing
As your students sequence the events in this story, use this list as a guide.
1. It is night on the farm.
2. The boy hears music coming from the barn.
3. The boy goes to the barn to see what is going on.
4. The scarecrow and the animals are having a barn dance.
5. The dance is over and the boy goes back to his house to go to bed.

#BK-272 Year-Round Literature • ©1999 Super Duper® Publications • 1-800-277-8737 • www.superduperinc.com

# Farm Articulation and Language Games

(The following games can be used with the articulation and vocabulary word list or the literature language questions.)

## Barn Game

Make copies of the barn pattern (page 158) on red or white construction paper. Cut out and laminate the barns. Place cards number side down on the table. After a student makes a sentence with a farm word containing his/her sound or answers a farm language question, the student may draw a barn. The number on the back is the number of points the student receives on the score sheet for the turn. The student with the most points wins.

### Team Approach

In order to win the game, the team must earn a designated number of points. For example, to win, the team must have 30 points by the end of the class.

## Puzzle Game

Photocopy, color, laminate, and cut the puzzles apart (page 159). Put each puzzle into a separate envelope. When playing, give each student a puzzle with all of the pieces facedown. After a student makes a sentence with a farm word containing his/her sound or answers a farm language question, the student may turn over one piece of his/her puzzle. The object is for each student to have his/her puzzle completely together by the end of class.

### Language Extension

After completing each puzzle, allow each student to describe the farm animal pictured. Talk about what the farm animal looks like, sounds like, what it does on the farm, the name of its baby, etc.

## Barrier Game

Photocopy, color, and laminate the farm scenes (page 160 and 162). Photocopy, color, cut out, and laminate farm objects (page 161). Separate the students using a tall box or therapy mirror. Give one team a completed scene. Give the other team the empty scene and objects. The team with the completed scene must describe to the other team where each object should be placed. The team placing objects is allowed to ask three questions in order to ensure proper placement. The object is for the team with the empty scene and objects to recreate the completed scene of the other team. The game is ideal for students working on language and listening skills or for those students who are at the sentence or conversation level of articulation therapy.

## Eggs in the Basket Game

Photocopy, color, cut out, and laminate the eggs (page 163). Turn the eggs facedown. After a student makes a sentence with a farm word containing his/her sound or answers a farm language question, the student chooses one egg card. If the egg has directions, the student must follow the directions. If the egg is blank, the student may keep the egg. The student with the most eggs at the end of the game is the winner.

### Team Approach

In order to win, the team must earn a designated number of eggs. For example, the team must have 15 eggs by the end of class to win.

## Parts of a Scarecrow Game

Photocopy, color, and laminate the scarecrow game board (page 164). Then, photocopy the following student sheet (page 165) for each student. (You may photocopy front and back to save paper and use the back side with the next therapy group.) Make a game die using a penny. Put a piece of masking tape on both sides and write a "2' on one side and a "3" on the other side with permanent ink.

Discuss the different parts of the scarecrow on the game board and tell the class that the goal is for each student to get each part to complete the scarecrow on the student sheet. Then, give each child a student sheet and a pencil. After a student makes a sentence with a farm word containing his/her sound or answers a farm language question, the student may flip the penny die, move the allotted spaces around the game board, and then draw the scarecrow part on the student sheet.

### Language Extension

After completing the scarecrow, discuss the purpose of the scarecrow and different types of crops the scarecrow protects.

# Barn Game

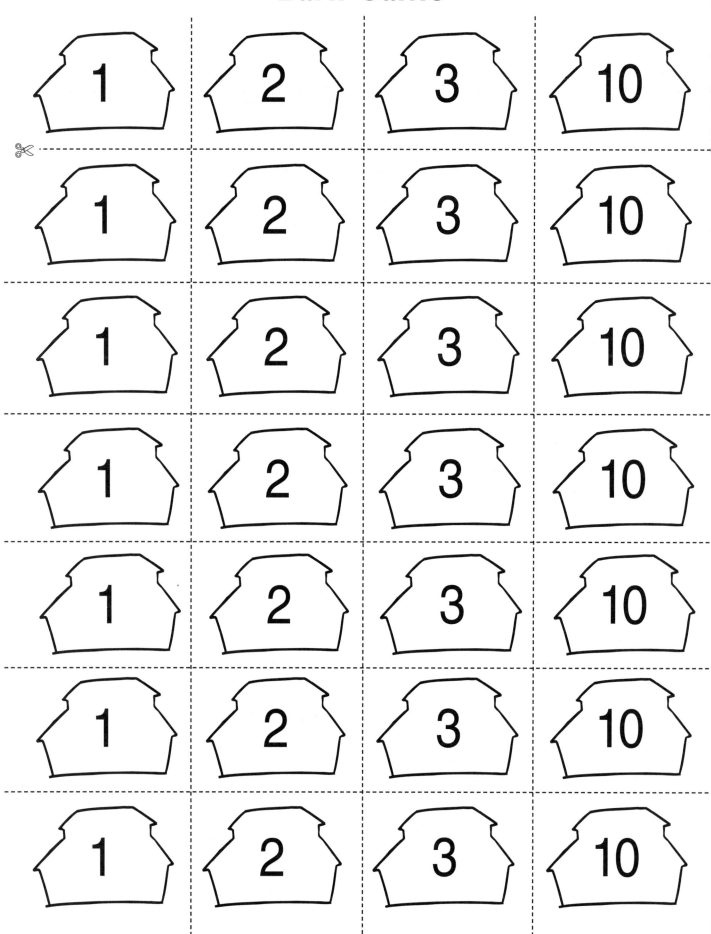

#BK-272  Year-Round Literature  •  ©1999 Super Duper® Publications  •  1-800-277-8737  •  www.superduperinc.com

# Puzzle Game

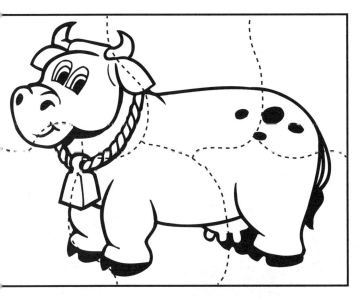

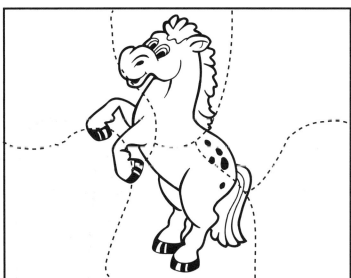

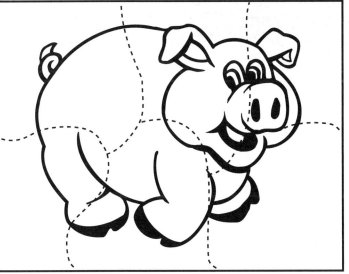

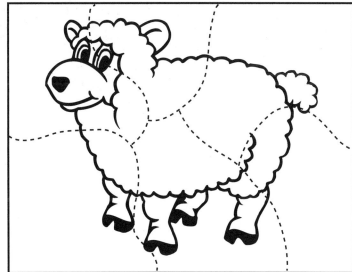

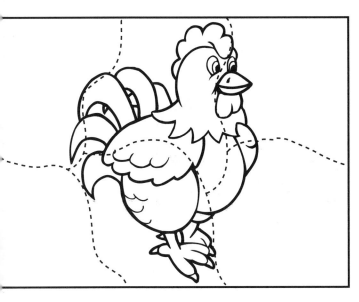

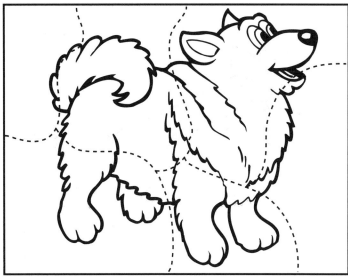

# Barrier Game

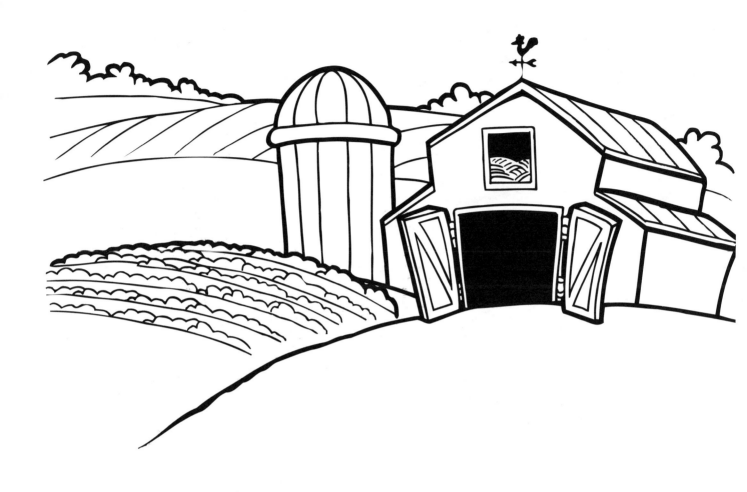

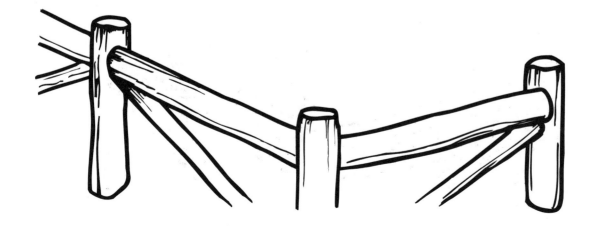

 #BK-272  Year-Round Literature  •  ©1999 Super Duper® Publications  •  1-800-277-8737  •  www.superduperinc.com

# Barrier Game

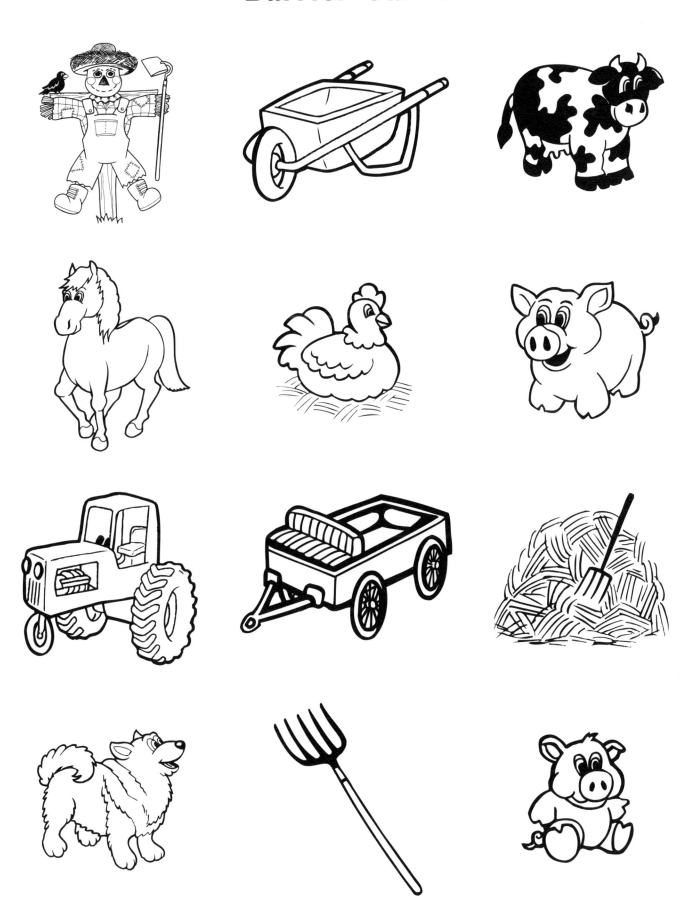

# Barrier Game

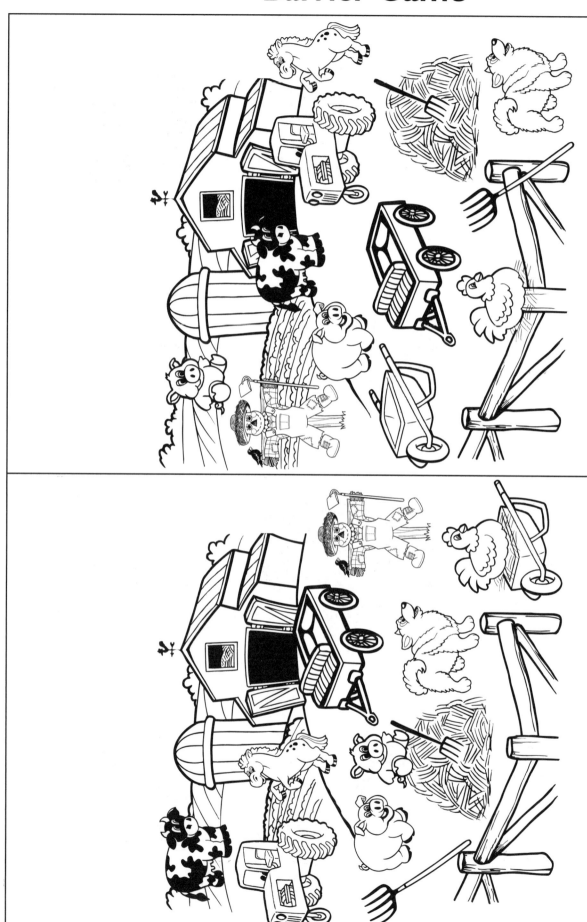

#BK-272  Year-Round Literature  •  ©1999 Super Duper® Publications  •  1-800-277-8737  •  www.superduperinc.com

# Eggs in the Basket Game

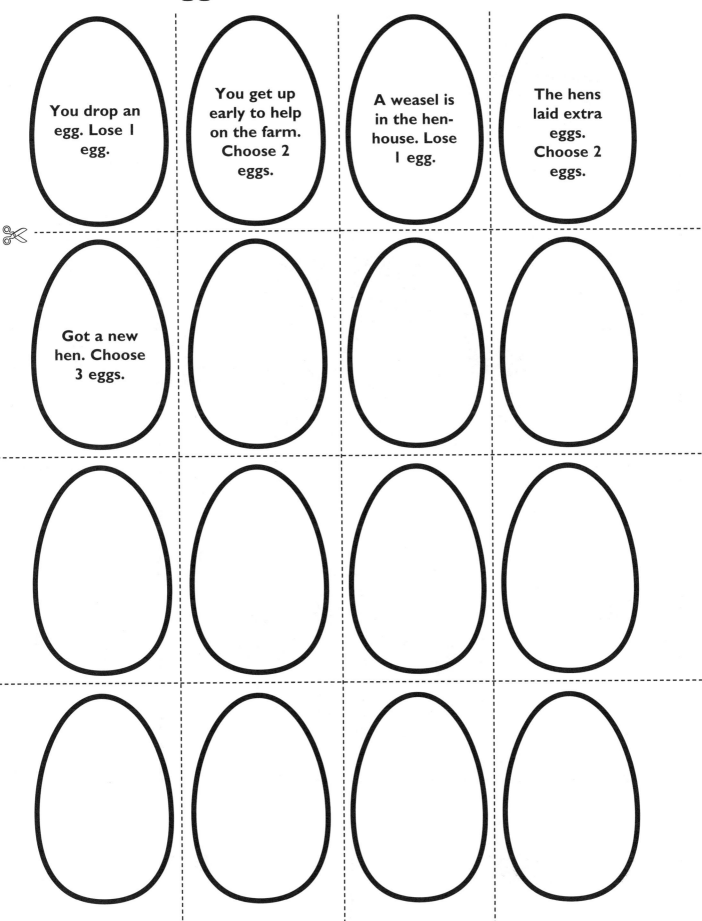

You drop an egg. Lose 1 egg.

You get up early to help on the farm. Choose 2 eggs.

A weasel is in the hen-house. Lose 1 egg.

The hens laid extra eggs. Choose 2 eggs.

Got a new hen. Choose 3 eggs.

# Parts of a Scarecrow Board Game

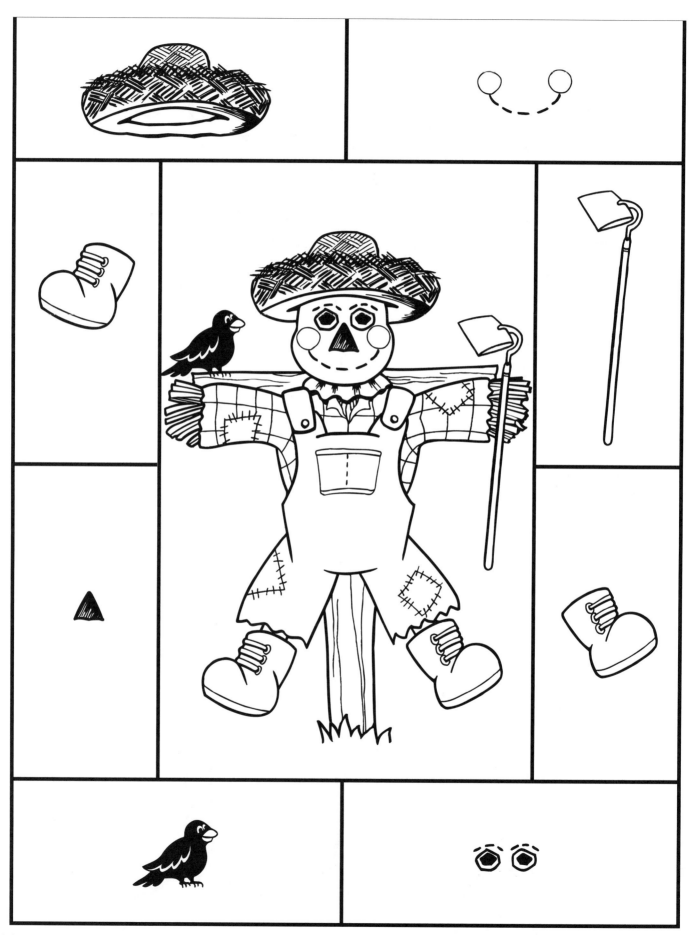

# Parts of a Scarecrow Student Sheet

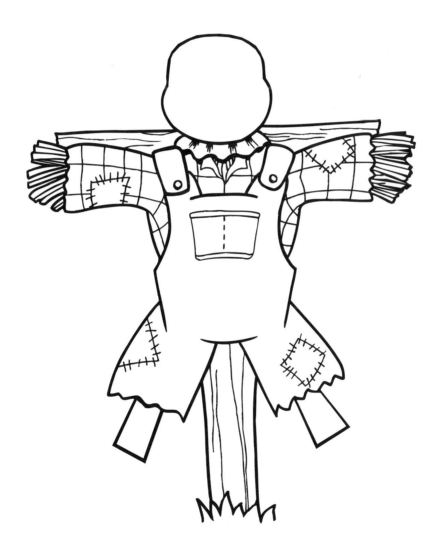

# Fill Your Barn with Good Speech

Write words with the _____ sound on the lines in the barn.
Make a sentence out loud using your good speech.

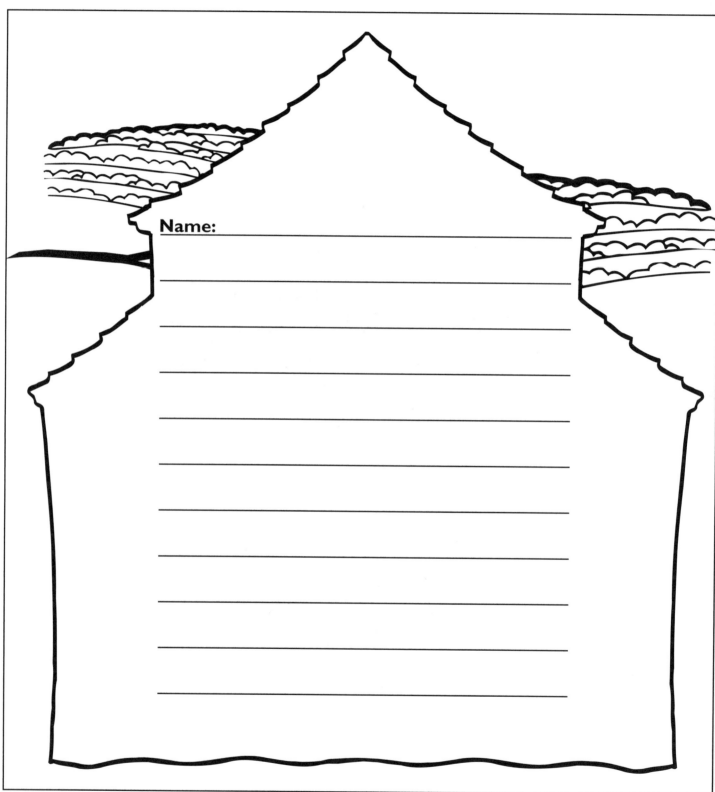

Name: _____

Name _____   Date _____

Speech-Language Pathologist          Helper's Signature

#BK-272 Year-Round Literature • ©1999 Super Duper® Publications • 1-800-277-8737 • www.superduperinc.com

# Adult and Baby Farm Animals

Look at the pictures below. Which pictures go together? Draw a line from one picture to the picture it goes with. Then, tell why the pictures go together using your good speech.

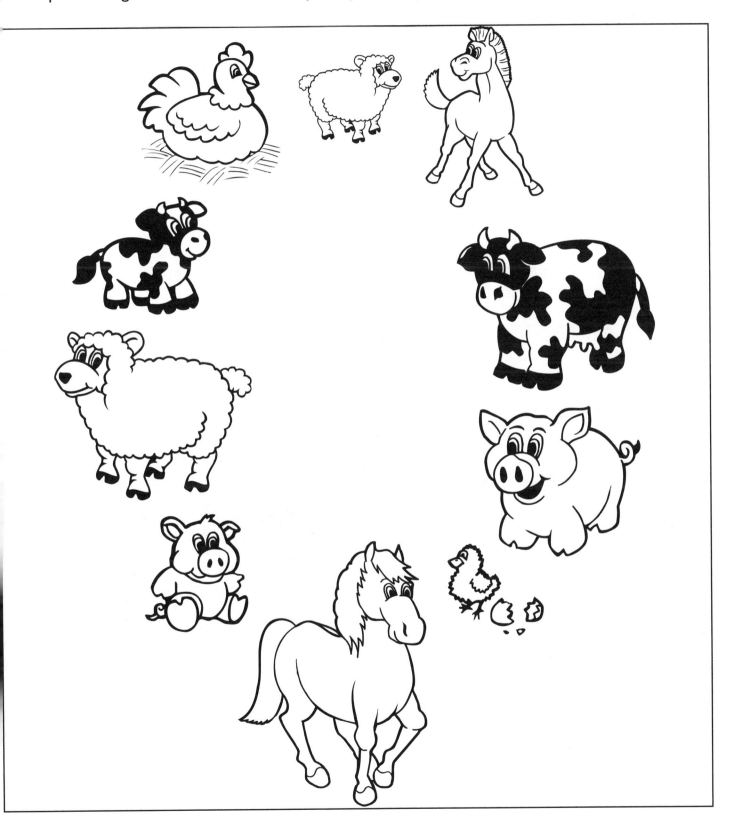

Name _____  Date _____

Speech-Language Pathologist                    Helper's Signature

#BK-272  Year-Round Literature  •  ©1999 Super Duper® Publications  •  1-800-277-8737  •  www.superduperinc.com

# Animal Homes

Write the names of three animals that live in each of the places shown below.

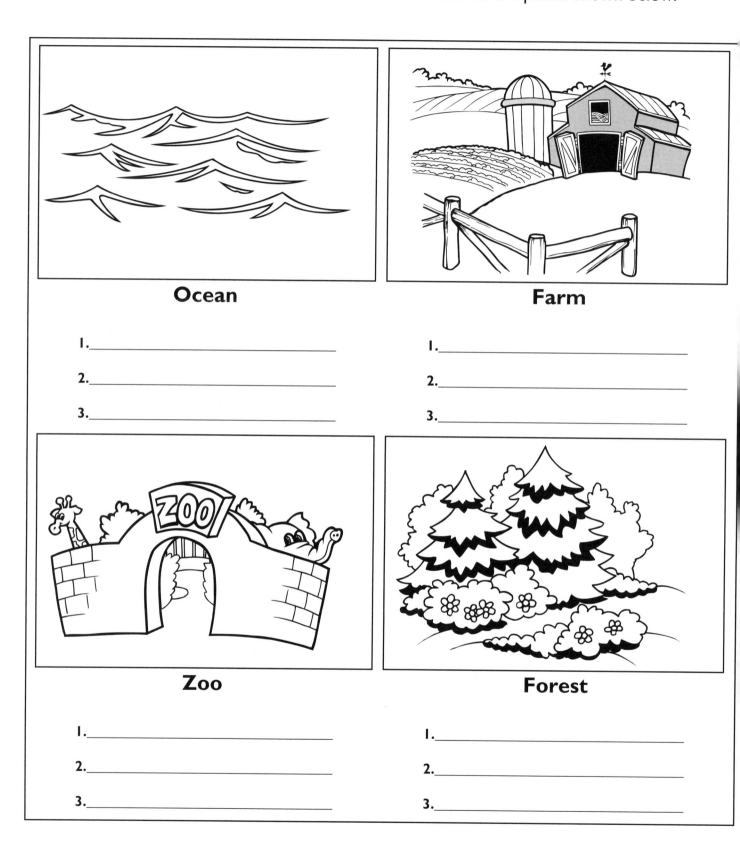

**Ocean**

1._____

2._____

3._____

**Farm**

1._____

2._____

3._____

**Zoo**

1._____

2._____

3._____

**Forest**

1._____

2._____

3._____

Name _____     Date _____

Speech-Language Pathologist                              Helper's Signature

#BK-272  Year-Round Literature  •  ©1999 Super Duper® Publications  •  1-800-277-8737  •  www.superduperinc.com

# Our Town

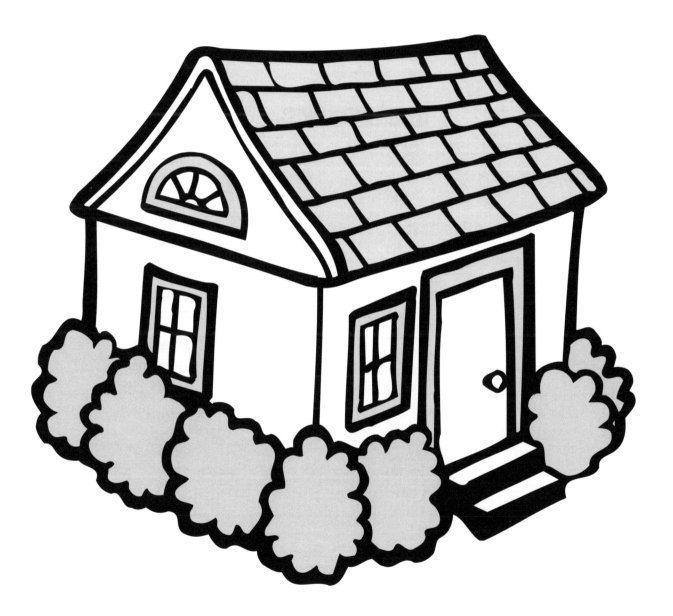

# Our Town Articulation & Vocabulary Word Lists

These word lists are a good resource for articulation and/or vocabulary building activities.

## /r/ and /r/ blends

### Initial
road
room
road sign
recycle
wreck

### Medial
tourist
supermarket
motorcycle
firefighter
railroad
restaurant

### Final
door
bus driver
car
police officer
police car
helicopter
neighbor
street sweeper
store
shoe store
clothing store
picnic shelter
skyscraper
teacher
river

### Blends
drug
street
traffic
tree
grass
bus driver
train
railroad tracks
truck
street sweeper
train station
drug store
grocery store
bridge
semi truck
freeway

playground
country
airport
airplane
garbage truck
billboard
apartment
park
parking lot
church
park bench
forklift
railroad tracks

## /s/ and /s/ blends

### Initial
city
subway
supermarket
semi truck
sailboat
soccer field
cinema

### Medial
police officer
gas pump
bicycle
motorcycle
baseball field
asphalt
recycle
sunset

### Final
house
grass
bus
railroad tracks
ambulance
apartments
fence
warehouse
cats

### Blends
street
stop sign
street sweeper

train station
grocery store
shoe store
clothing store
drug store
gas station
swing set
slide
skyscraper
school
station wagon
school bus
stadium
smoke stack
statue
toy store
jewelry store
taxi
hospital
restaurant
tourist
basketball court

## /z/

### Initial
zoo

### Medial
museum
newspaper

### Final
trees
neighbors
clouds
dogs
sunrise
neon signs
noise

## /l/ and /l/ blends

### Initial
light
lake
library

#BK-272  Year-Round Literature  •  ©1999 Super Duper® Publications  •  1-800-277-8737  •  www.superduperinc.com

# Our Town Articulation & Vocabulary Word Lists (Cont.)

## /l/ and /l/ blends cont.

### Medial
railroad tracks
police officer
police car
ambulance
helicopter
billboard
forklift
pollution
sailboat
telephone pole

### Final
city hall
wheel
hospital
hotel
basketball

### Blends
people
rollerbladers
airplane
clothing store
slide
playground
flag
flagpole
clouds
bicycle
motorcycle
jewelry store
windshield wipers
rollerbladers
plot
capitol building
shelter
office building
railroad tracks

## /k/ and /k/ blends

### Initial
country
car
condominiums
capitol building
cats
cab

### Medial
helicopter
picnic shelter
soccer field
electric poles

### Final
traffic
railroad track
work
fire truck
garbage truck
park
lake
bank
truck
sidewalk
honk
gas tank
dock
semi truck

### Blends
clothing store
clouds
skyscraper
school
school bus
concrete
bicycle
recycle
motorcycle
basketball court
taxi
supermarket

## /g/ and /g/ blends

### Initial
gas station
gas pump

### Medial
tugboat

### Final
flag

### Blends
grass
playground
grocery store

## /th/

### Initial
theater

### Medial
weather
clothing store

## /sh/

### Initial
shoe store
shelter
shopping
shop
shopping mall

### Medial
windshield wiper
bus station
train station
grocery store
gas station
station wagon
pollution
police station

### Final
trash

## /ch/

### Initial
chimney

### Medial
teacher
preacher

### Final
park bench
church

# Our Town Articulation & Vocabulary Word Lists (Con

## /m/ and /m/ blends

### Initial
mall

### Medial
apartments
condominiums
supermarket
semi truck
pavement
chimney
cinema

### Final
room
museum
stadium

### Blends
gas pump
smokestack
ambulance
pharmacy

## /p/ and /p/ blends

### Initial
people
police officer
police car
pilot
park
pond
park bench
picnic shelter
pole
pollution
power lines
pavements
pets
parking lot

### Medial
windshield wipers
helicopter
airport
street sweeper
apartments
capitol building
skyscraper
shopping

### Final
bus stop
gas pump
flower shop

### Blends
airplane
playground
hospital
people

## /b/ and /b/ blends

### Initial
boat
barge
birds
bus
bus stop
bus driver
building
bench
bicycle

### Medial
sailboat
neighborhood
neighbors
harbor
tugboat
subway
ambulance
garbage truck
billboard
baseball
basketball

### Final
cab

### Blends
bridge
library

## /f/ and /f/ blends

### Initial
fire truck
fire station
fire hydrant
fence
ferry

fountain
pharmacy
factory

### Medial
traffic
firefighter
office building
asphalt

### Blends
flight attendant
freeway
flag
flagpole
freight train
freighter
flower shop
forklift

## /v/

### Medial
river
elevator

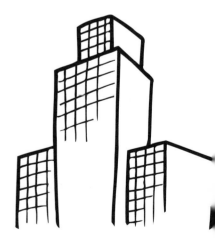

#BK-272  Year-Round Literature  •  ©1999 Super Duper® Publications  •  1-800-277-8737  •  www.superduperinc.com

# Vocabulary Pictures

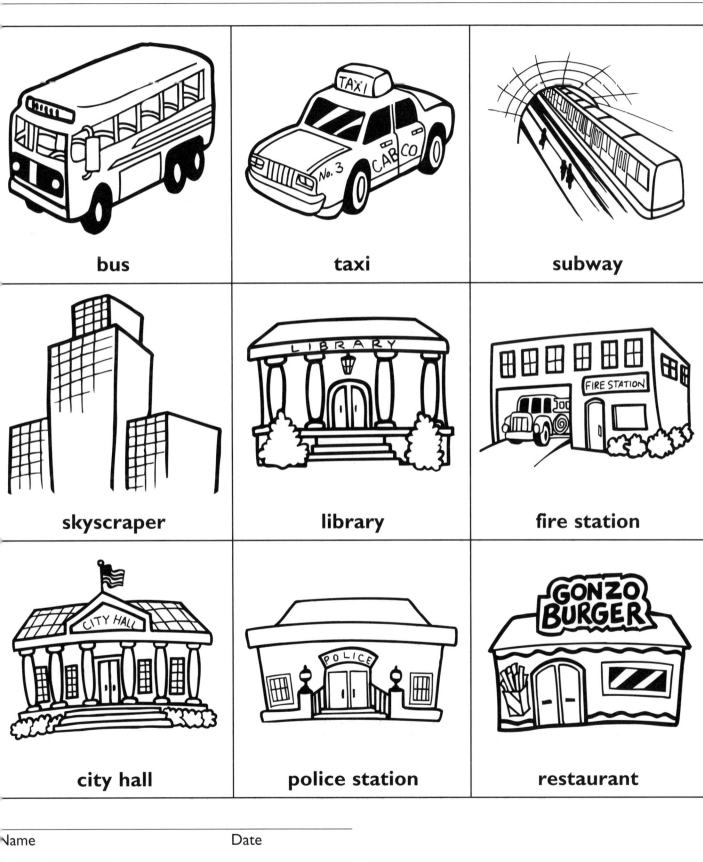

bus

taxi

subway

skyscraper

library

fire station

city hall

police station

restaurant

# Vocabulary Pictures

**Instructions:** _____

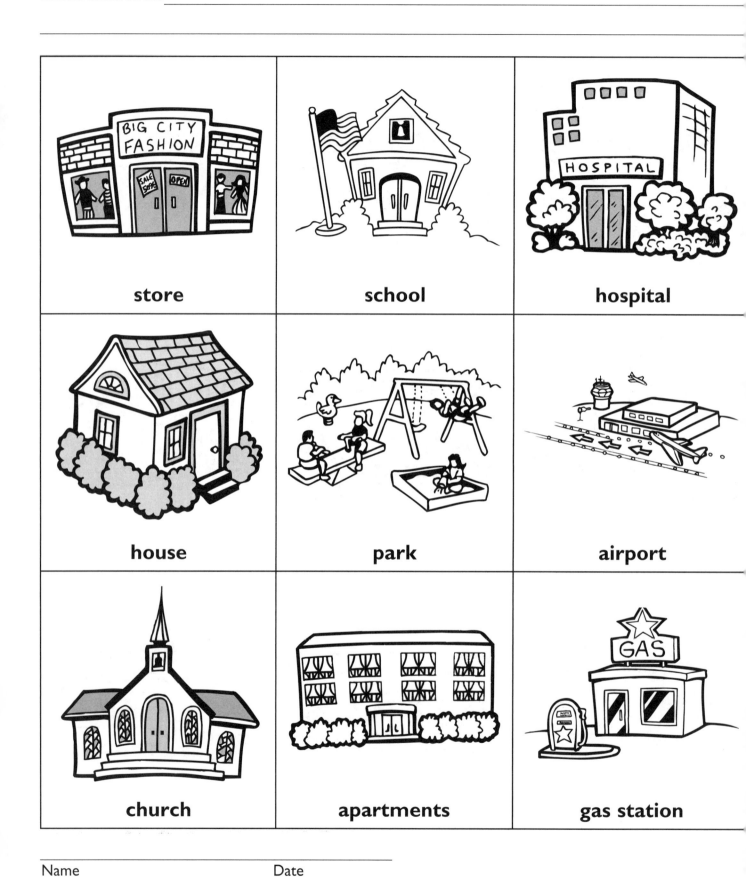

| | | |
|---|---|---|
| store | school | hospital |
| house | park | airport |
| church | apartments | gas station |

Name _____  Date _____

# Vocabulary Pictures

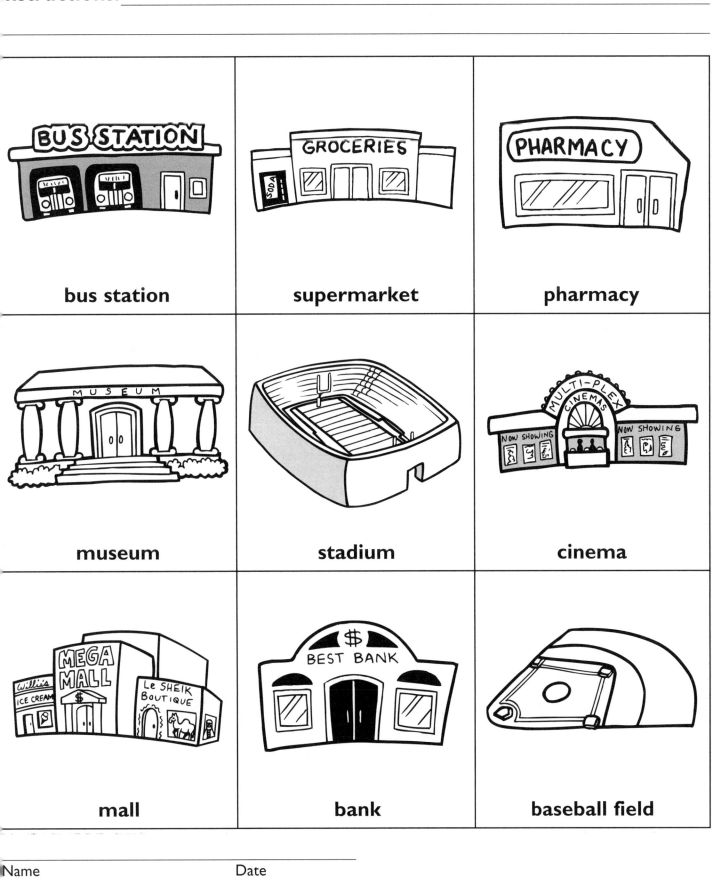

| | | |
|---|---|---|
| bus station | supermarket | pharmacy |
| museum | stadium | cinema |
| mall | bank | baseball field |

Name _____ Date _____

Speech-Language Pathologist _____ Helper's Signature _____

#BK-272  Year-Round Literature  •  ©1999 Super Duper® Publications  •  1-800-277-8737  •  www.superduperinc.com

175

# Story Pattern

Name: _____

_____

_____

_____

_____

_____

_____

_____

_____

_____

_____

_____

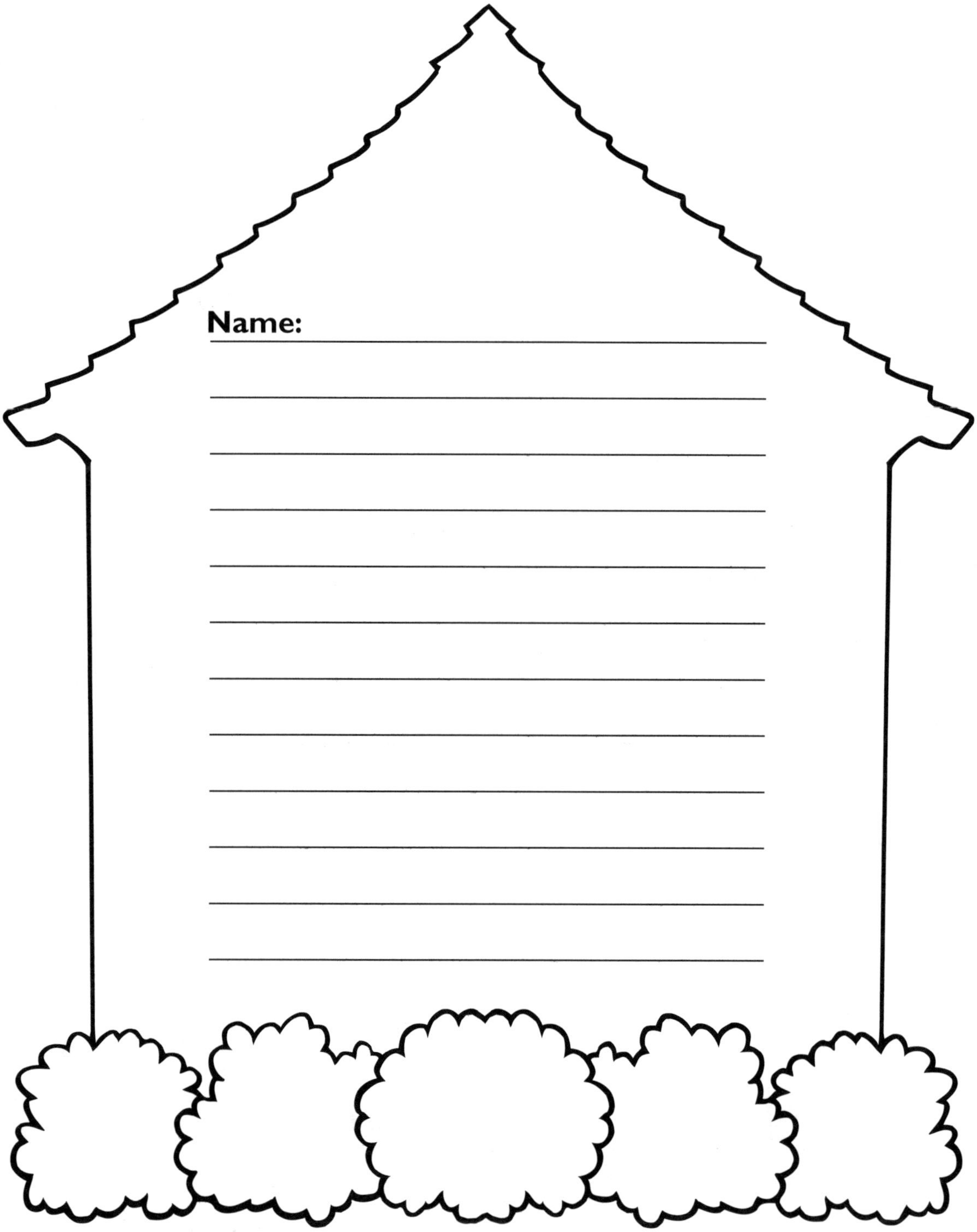

Name _____          Date _____

Speech-Language Pathologist          Helper's Signature

# Me on the Map
## by Joan Sweeney

This is a book that takes the reader from a girl's house to her street, to her town, to her state, to her country, and to her planet. For each place, the girl gives a short description and shows a map. The story line is based on the theme that no matter where you live, you have a special place to call your own.

**Language Expansion:** The following questions can be used to address students' recall of this book

# Definition
1. What is a map?
2. What is a street?
3. What is a town?
4. What is a state?
5. What is a country?

# Function
1. What is a map used for?
2. What is a room used for?
3. What is a house used for?
4. What is a street used for?
5. What is a town used for?

# Category
1. Name three rooms of a house.
2. Name three streets.
3. Name three states.
4. Name three countries.
5. Name three things you can do with a map.

# Description
1. Tell me three things about your room.
2. Tell me three things about your house.
3. Tell me three things about your street.
4. Tell me three things about your town.
5. Tell me three things about your coun-

# Vocabulary
Make a sentence using the following words.
1. map
2. town
3. state
4. country
5. Earth

# Rhyming
Name a rhyming word for each word below.
1. map
2. place
3. town
4. state

# Sequencing
As your students sequence the events in this story, use this list as a guide.
1. The book talks about a girl in her house on her street.
2. The book talks about the town and the state that the girl lives in.
3. The book talks about the country the girl lives in.
4. The book talks about the girl's planet.
5. The book says that no matter where you live, you have a special place that is all your own.

# The Adventures of Taxi Dog
## by Debra and Sal Barracca

This is a story about a homeless dog that is picked up and taken home by a taxi driver named Jim. Maxi, the dog, rides around each day in the taxi with Jim. They have many adventures as they drive around the city.

**Language Expansion:** The following questions can be used to address students' recall of this book or to expand upon concepts addressed in this book.

## Definition
1. What is a taxi?
2. What is a pound (dog pound)?
3. What is a scarf?
4. What is a taxi fare?
5. What is an airport?

## Function
1. What is a taxi for?
2. What is food for?
3. What is a plate for?
4. What is a home for?
5. What is a hospital for?

## Category
1. Name three things you might see in a city.
2. Name three parts of a taxi.
3. Name three parts of a dog.
4. Name three things at an airport.
5. Name three things you can do at a circus.

## Description
1. Tell me three things about a dog.
2. Tell me three things about a taxi.
3. Tell me three things about a city.
4. Tell me three things about an airport.
5. Tell me three things about a circus.

## Vocabulary
Make a sentence using the following words.
1. park
2. home
3. building
4. circus
5. passenger

## Rhyming
Name a rhyming word for each word below
1. day
2. dark
3. seat
4. head
5. town

## Sequencing
As your students sequence the events in this story, use this list as a guide.
1. Maxi is a dog without a home.
2. Jim found Maxi and took him home.
3. Now they ride around together in Jim's taxi.
4. They drive around the city and pick up a singer, a man and a lady who have a baby, people from the airport, some clowns, and a chimp.
5. At the end of their day, they earn their pay and go home together.

#BK-272  Year-Round Literature  •  ©1999 Super Duper® Publications  •  1-800-277-8737  •  www.superduperinc.com

# Secret Place
## by Eve Bunting

This is a book about a little boy who lives in a busy city. The city is loud and crowded, but the little boy has found a secret place. The secret place is a quiet spot along a river where one might even see some ducklings.

**Language Expansion:** The following questions can be used to address students' recall of this book or to expand upon concepts addressed in this book.

## Definition
1. What is a city?
2. What is a freeway?
3. What is a river?
4. What are binoculars?
5. What are ducklings?

## Function
1. What is a railroad track used for?
2. What is a smokestack used for?
3. What is a forklift used for?
4. What is a telephone pole used for?
5. What is a chimney used for?

## Category
1. Name three things you might see on a city street.
2. Name three animals that the boy found at the river.
3. Name three buildings that might be in a city.
4. Name three noises that you might hear in a city.
5. Name three things that you might do in a city.

## Description
1. Tell me three things about a city.
2. Tell me three things about a river.
3. Tell me three things about the secret place.
4. Tell me three things about binoculars.
5. Tell me three things about ducklings.

## Vocabulary
Make a sentence using the following words.
1. freeway
2. warehouse
3. telephone and electric poles
4. wilderness
5. traffic

## Rhyming
Name a rhyming word for each word below.
1. track
2. street
3. phone
4. pole
5. noise

## Sequencing
As your students sequence the events in this story, use this list as a guide.
1. A little boy lives in a very crowded and busy city.
2. In the heart of the city is a secret place by the river.
3. Only a few people know about the secret place by the river.
4. There are egrets, ducks, coyotes, and possums at the secret place.
5. The secret place is a very special place that the little boy never wants to change.

# Our Town Articulation and Language Games

(The following games can be used with the articulation and vocabulary word list or the literature language questions.)

## Building a Town Game

Make one copy of the building pattern (page 181) for each student. Color the buildings, cut them apart, and laminate them. Tell the students that you are going to build a town. Each student must get a town hall, a police station, a fire station, a store, and a library by the end of class. After a student makes a sentence with a town word containing his/her sound or answers a town language question, the student may reach into the bag and pull out one building. (If the child does not have the building drawn, he/she may keep it. If the child does have the building drawn, he/she must put it back and wait for the next turn.) Whoever collects all of the buildings first is the winner.

### Team Approach

In order to win the game, each team member must collect all six buildings by the end of class.

## Going to the Shopping Mall Game

Make one copy of the shopping mall board (page 182) for each student. Color, cut out, and laminate each game board. Color, cut out, and laminate the direction cards. The object of the game is to get from home to the shopping mall. After a student makes a sentence with a town word containing his/her sound or answers a town language question, the student may choose a direction card. The direction card will tell the student to move forward a certain number of steps, backward a certain number of steps, or to remain in place. The student who gets to the shopping mall first is the winner of the game.

### Language Extension

After completing the game, ask the students to brainstorm the things they might see in a shopping mall. Then, discuss ways to get to the mall and places that you would pass on the way to the shopping mall.

## Taxi Game

Photocopy the taxi pattern (page 183) on yellow construction paper, cut it out, and laminate. Turn the cards facedown. After a student makes a sentence with a town word containing his/her sound or answers a town language question, the student chooses one taxi card. If the taxi has directions, the student must follow the directions. If the taxi is blank, the student may keep the taxi. The student with the most taxis at the end of the game is the winner.

### Team Approach

In order to win the game, the team must earn a designated number of taxis. For example, the team must have 15 taxis by the end of class to win.

## Bus Game

Photocopy the bus pattern (page 184) on yellow or blue construction paper. Cut out and laminate the buses. Place buses number side down on the table. After a student makes a sentence with a town word containing his/her sound or answers a town language question, the student may draw a bus. The number on the back is the number of points the student received on the score sheet for the turn. The student with the most points wins.

### Team Approach

In order to win the game, the team must earn a certain number of points. For example, the team must have 30 points by the end of class to win.

## City Matching Game

Photocopy two copies of each of the city objects (page 185). Color, cut out, and laminate the city object cards. Lay the cards facedown and allow each student to turn over two cards. If the cards don't match, the student must choose one of the cards to name and describe using good speech and language and then put both cards facedown. If the cards match, the student must tell about the city object by naming it and describing it using good speech and language. Then, the student may keep the matching pair. Continue taking turns until all of the city objects have been matched. The student with the most matches wins.

### Team Approach

In order to win the game, the team must be able to match all of the city objects by the end of the therapy session.

 #BK-272 Year-Round Literature • ©1999 Super Duper® Publications • 1-800-277-8737 • www.superduperinc.com

# Building a Town Game

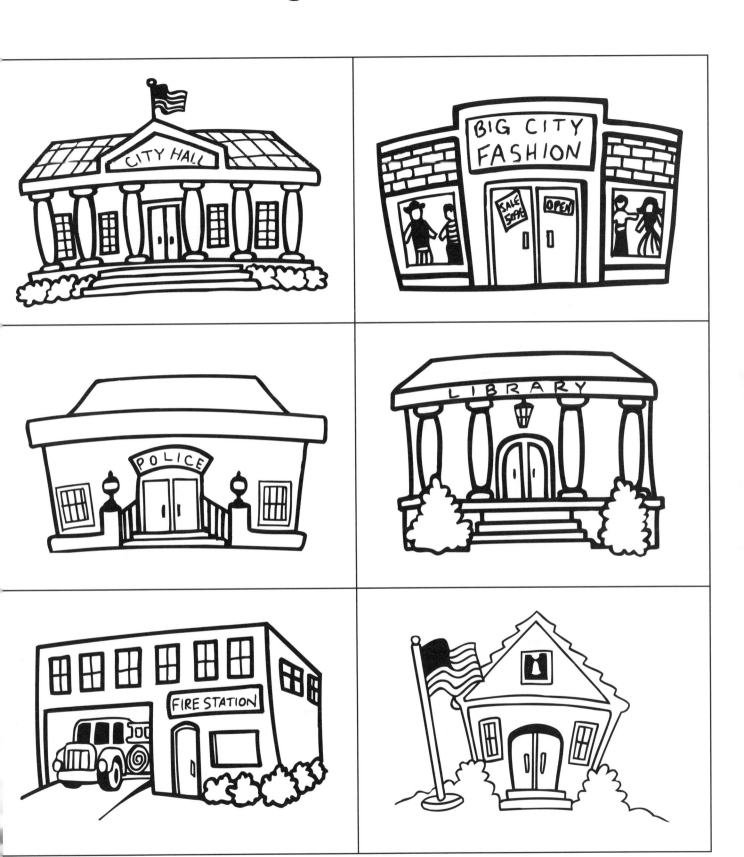

# Going to the Shopping Mall

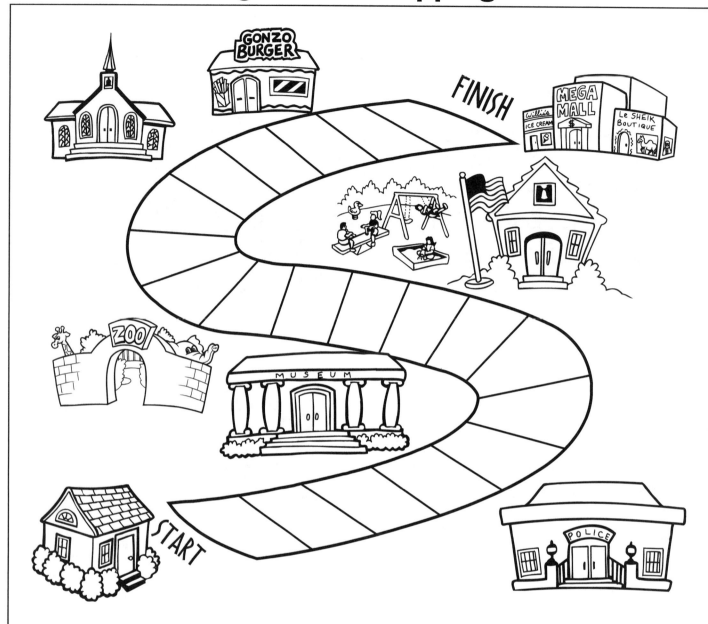

| You remember to wear your seat belt. Go forward 3 steps. | Ran out of gas. Go backward 3 steps. | The traffic light is green. Go forward 2 steps. | Rain slows down traffic. Go backward 2 steps. |
|---|---|---|---|
| You have a full tank of gas. Go forward 1 step. | You forgot your money. Go backward 1 step. | Traffic jam on the interstate. Stay where you are. | You see someone you know. Go forward 1 step. |

 #BK-272   Year-Round Literature  •  ©1999 Super Duper® Publications  •  1-800-277-8737  •  www.superduperinc.com

# Taxi Game

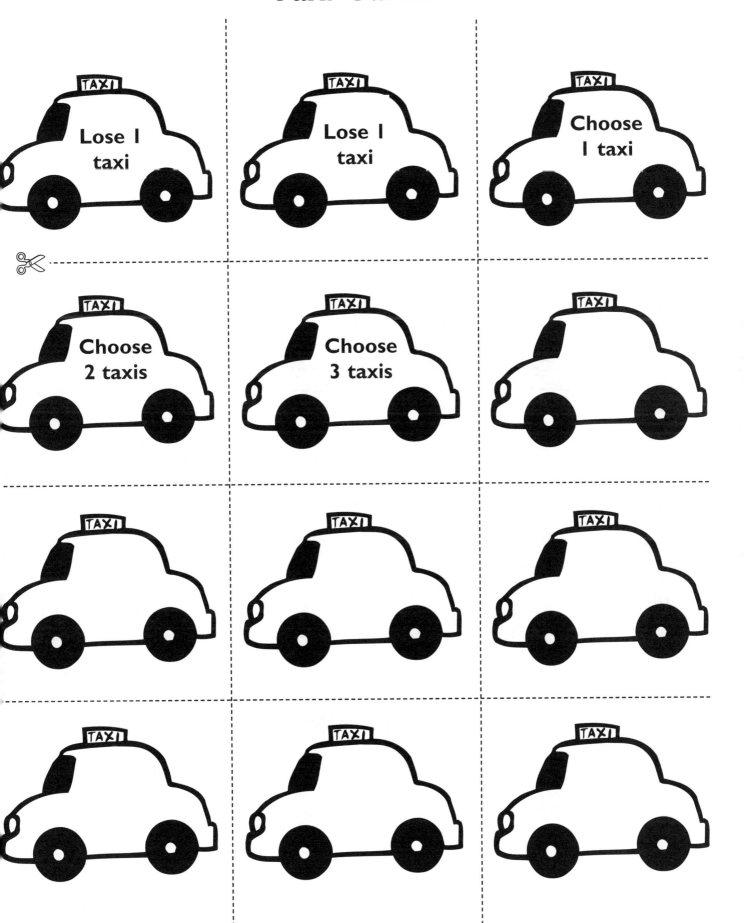

Lose 1 taxi

Lose 1 taxi

Choose 1 taxi

Choose 2 taxis

Choose 3 taxis

# Bus Game

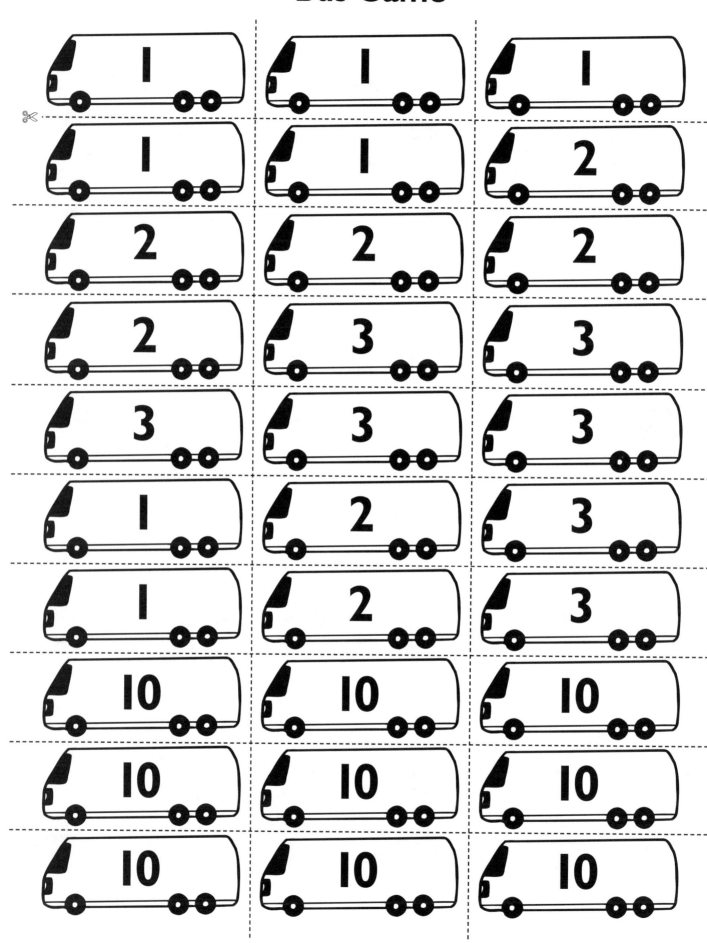

#BK-272  Year-Round Literature  •  ©1999 Super Duper® Publications  •  1-800-277-8737  •  www.superduperinc.com

# City Matching Game

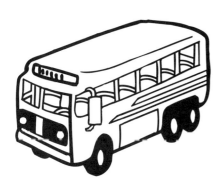

**bus**

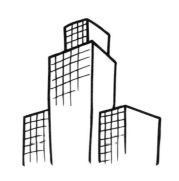

**skyscraper**

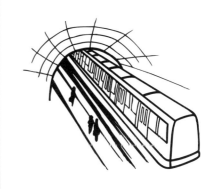

**subway**

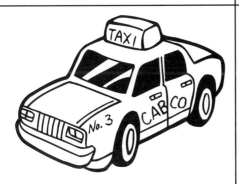

**taxi**

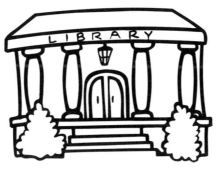

**library**

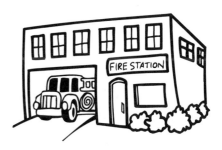

**fire station**

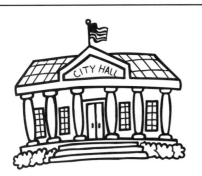

**city hall**

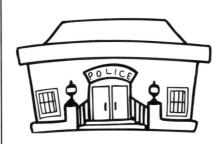

**police station**

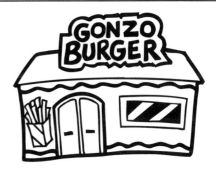

**restaurant**

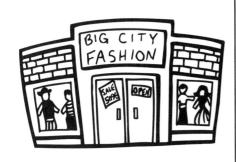

**store**

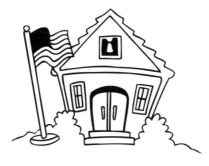

**school**

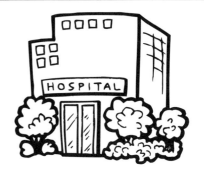

**hospital**

# Building Good Speech

Write words with the _____ sound in each building. Then, make a sentence with each word out loud using your good speech.

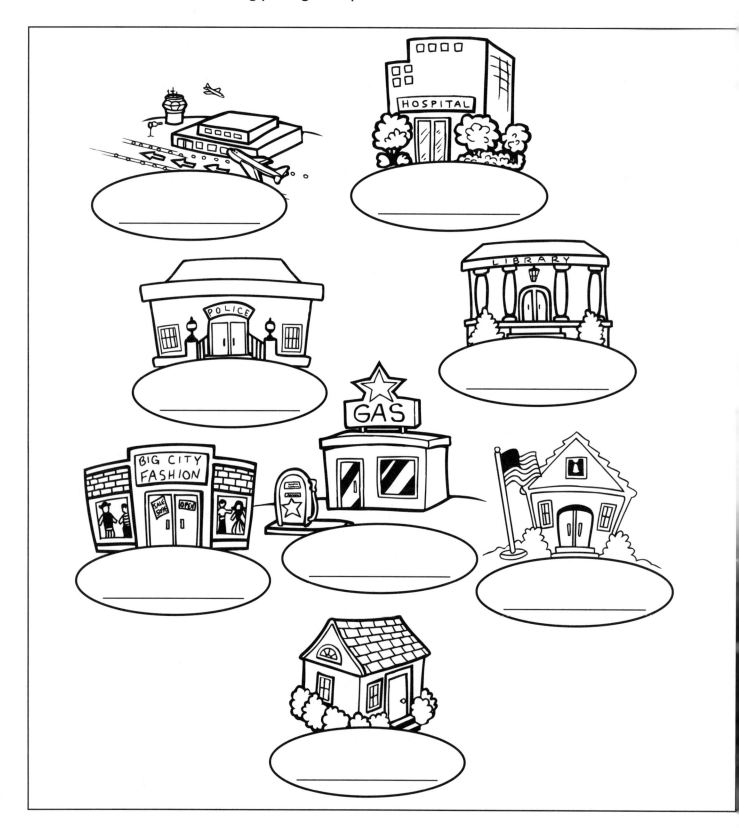

Name _____     Date _____

Speech-Language Pathologist                          Helper's Signature

#BK-272  Year-Round Literature  •  ©1999 Super Duper® Publications  •  1-800-277-8737  •  www.superduperinc.com

# Around Town

Look at the pictures below. Which pictures go together? Draw a line from one picture to the picture it goes with. Then, tell why the pictures go together using your good speech.

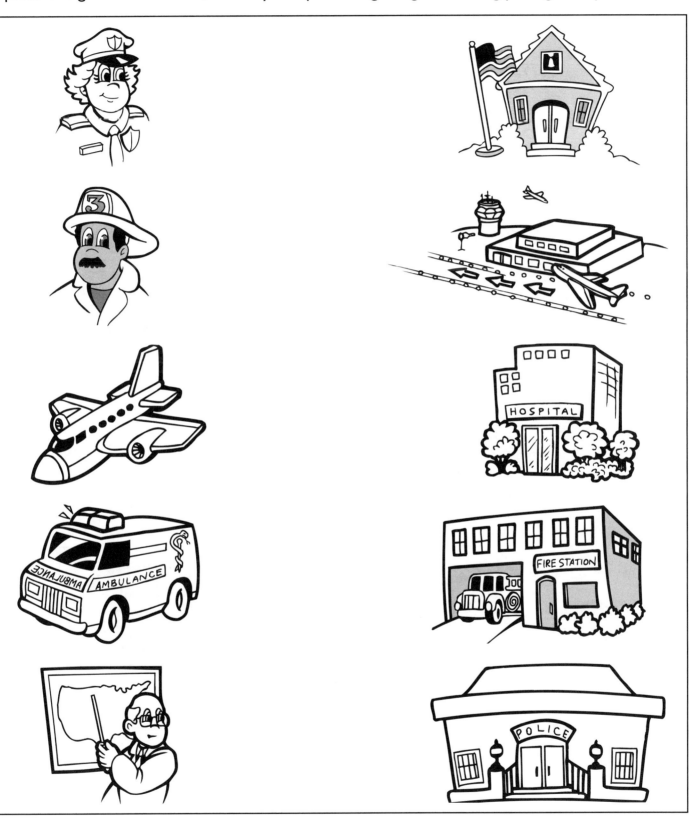

Name _____  Date _____

# Places to Go!

Towns have many places to go. Look at each picture below. Using the words in the box below, write the name of each town place on the line provided. Then, tell what you might do at each place using your good speech.

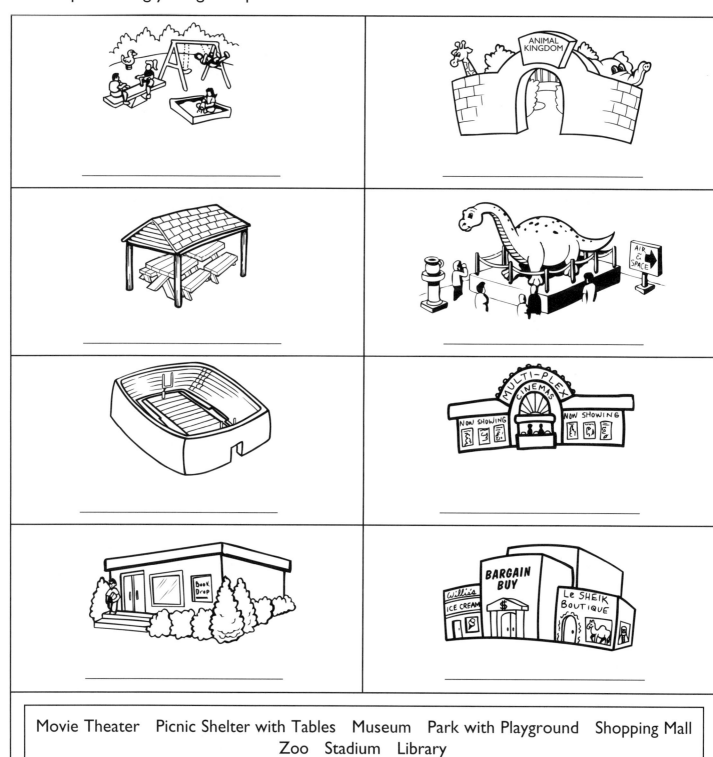

Movie Theater   Picnic Shelter with Tables   Museum   Park with Playground   Shopping Mall
Zoo   Stadium   Library

Name _____     Date _____

Speech-Language Pathologist          Helper's Signature

188          #BK-272  Year-Round Literature • ©1999 Super Duper® Publications • 1-800-277-8737 • www.superduperinc.com

# Ocean

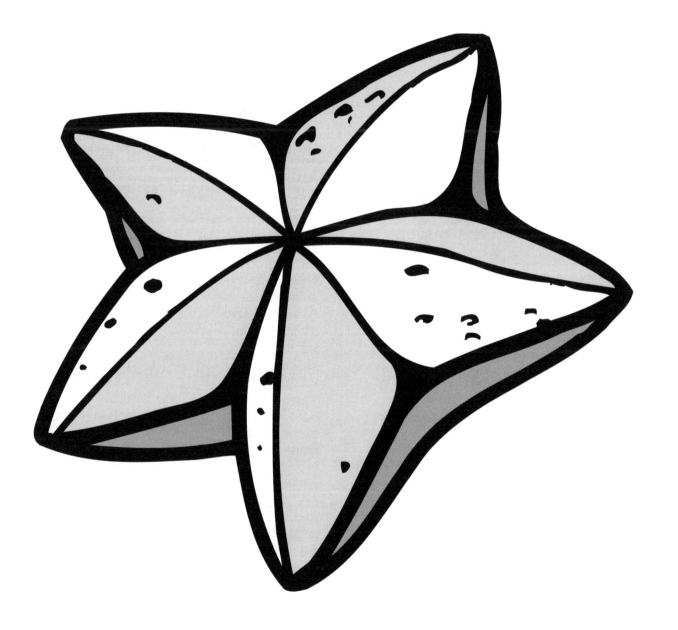

# Ocean Articulation & Vocabulary Word Lists

These word lists are a good resource for articulation and/or vocabulary building activities.

## /r/ and /r/ blends

### Initial
rainbow fish
reef

### Medial
stingray
starfish
barracuda
coral reef
sea urchin
butterfly fish
Arctic Ocean
submarine
The Red Sea
porpoise

### Final
lobster
anchor
water
oyster
sea otter
ocean liner
flounder
sand dollar
oceanographer
scuba diver

### Blends
crab
shrimp
sunscreen
oceanographer
scuba diver
walrus
hammerhead shark
shark
snorkeling
seahorse
sunburn
swordfish
lifeguard
turtle
iceberg

## /s/ and /s/ blends

### Initial
seal
sailboat
sand
seashell
sand bucket
sunbathing
suntan
sunburn
seaweed
sea otter
sea gull
sink
sea urchin
submarine
surfing
sand dollar

### Medial
Pacific Ocean
iceberg
bathing suit
sunglasses

### Final
octopus
walrus
porpoise
platypus
sand dunes
seahorse

### Blends
stingray
snorkeling
starfish
squid
swim
snail
lobster
oyster
scuba diver
sponge
swordfish
school of fish
seahorse
sandcastle
sunglasses
deep sea fishing

## /z/

### Initial
zoo

### Final
gills
fins
snails
sandals
sea lions
seals
squids
seashells
sand dunes

## /l/ and /l/ blends

### Initial
lobster
lifeguard

### Medial
jellyfish
beluga whale
sailboat
Atlantic Ocean
suntan lotion
sea lion
walrus
school of fish
platypus
ocean liner
ocean lettuce
scallops

### Final
beach ball
seal
whale
eel
coral
sea turtle
sea gull
coral
sandcastle
snail

### Blends
blue whale
flip-flops
float

butterfly fish
platypus
plankton
shovel
sandals
gills
sand dollar
killer whale
seashells

## /k/ and /k/ blends

### Initial
coral
catfish

### Medial
anchor
bucket
sand bucket
barracuda
sandcastle

### Final
shark
sink

### Blends
crab
sunscreen
squid
school of fish
scallops
scuba diving
snorkeling
octopus

## /g/ and /g/ blends

### Initial
gills
goldfish

### Medial
lifeguard
tugboat

### Blends
sunglasses
sea gull

#BK-272  Year-Round Literature • ©1999 Super Duper® Publications • 1-800-277-8737 • www.superduperinc.com

# Ocean Articulation & Vocabulary Word Lists (Cont.)

## /th/

### Initial
thermometer
three-spined
  stickleback

### Medial
sunbathing
warm weather
stormy weather
windy weather

## /sh/ and /sh/ blends

### Initial
shark
shovel
ship

### Medial
ocean
Pacific Ocean
Atlantic Ocean
suntan lotion
deep sea fishing
fish net
seashore
ocean liner
sunshine
oceanographer
seashell

### Final
jellyfish
starfish
sunfish
swordfish
school of fish

### Blends
shrimp

## /ch/

### Initial
channel catfish

### Medial
sea urchin
beach ball

### Final
beach
catch

## /m/ and /m/ blends

### Initial
manatee
motorboat

### Medial
hammerhead shark
hermit crab
submarine

### Final
swim

### Blends
shrimp

## /p/ and /p/ blends

### Initial
Pacific Ocean
puffer fish
pelican

### Medial
octopus
deep sea fishing

### Final
ship
scallop

### Blends
platypus
plankton
sponge

## /b/ and /b/ blends

### Initial
beluga whale
butterfly fish
bucket
bathing suit
barracuda
beach

### Medial
beach ball
scuba diver

sailboat
sand bucket
sun bathing
sunburn
rainbow fish
submarine
surfboard

### Final
crab

### Blends
blue whale
lobster

## /f/ and /f/ blends

### Initial
fish net

### Medial
dolphin
jellyfish
starfish
deep sea fishing
puffer fish

### Blends
float
flounder
flip flops
surfing
surf board

## /v/ and /v/ blends

### Medial
diver

### Final
wave

### Blends
shovel

# Vocabulary Pictures

**Instructions:** _____

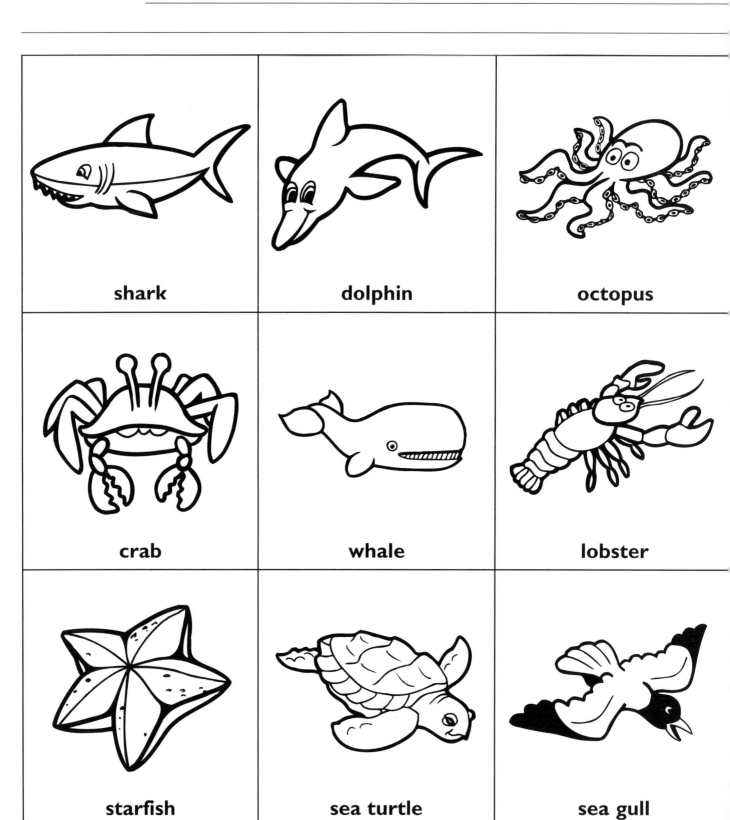

shark

dolphin

octopus

crab

whale

lobster

starfish

sea turtle

sea gull

Name _____  Date _____

Speech-Language Pathologist          Helper's Signature

# Vocabulary Pictures

| | | |
|---|---|---|
| seahorse | stingray | coral |
| seaweed | oyster | sailboat |
| flip-flops | wave | sunscreen |

# Vocabulary Pictures

**Instructions:** _____

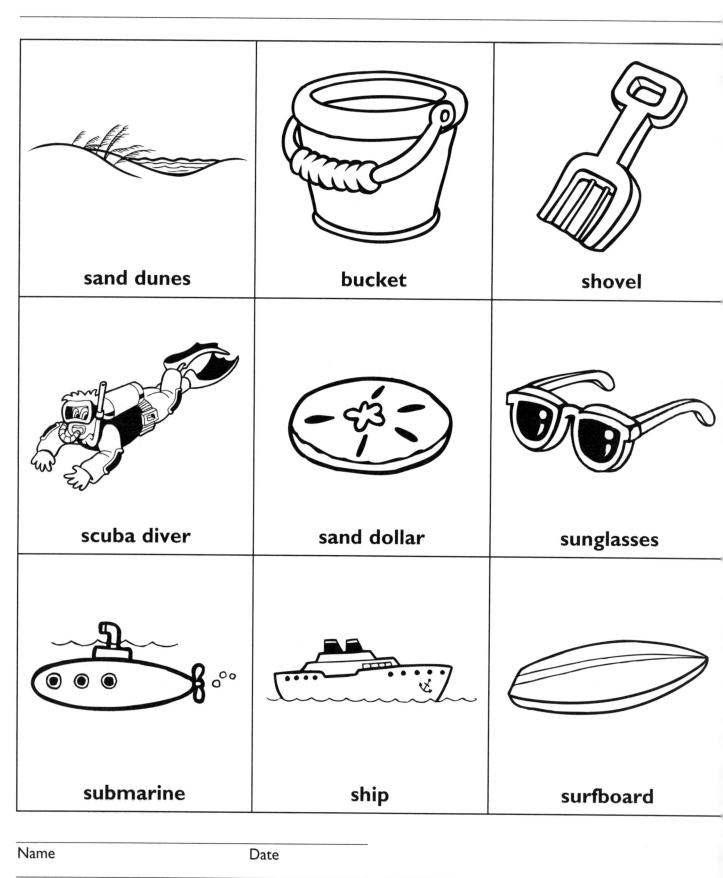

| | | |
|---|---|---|
| sand dunes | bucket | shovel |
| scuba diver | sand dollar | sunglasses |
| submarine | ship | surfboard |

Name _____     Date _____

# Story Pattern

**Name:** _____

_____

_____

_____

_____

_____

_____

_____

_____

_____

_____

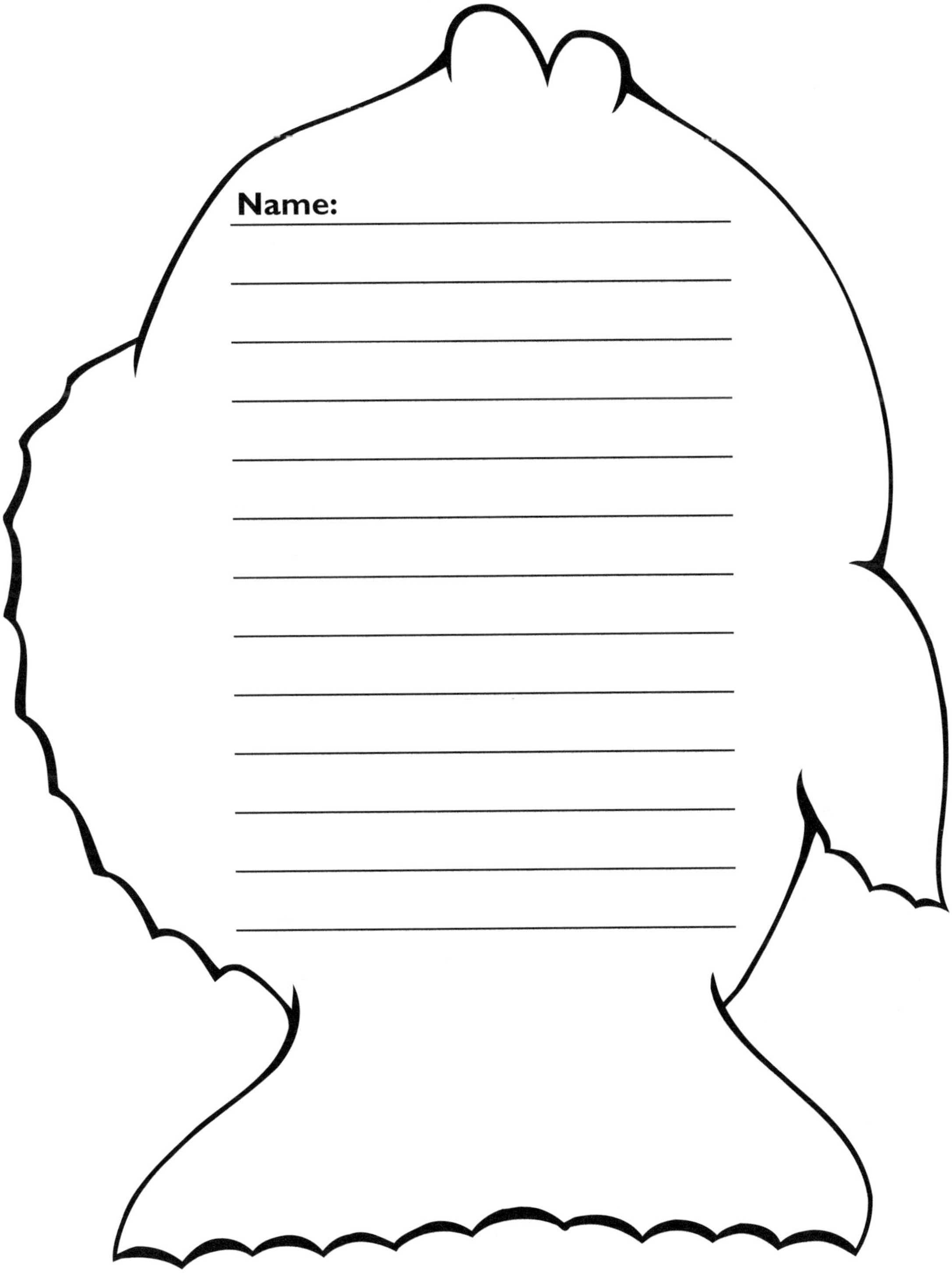

Name

Date

Speech-Language Pathologist

Helper's Signature

# Big Al

## by Andrew Clements

Big Al is a big fish who looks quite different from all of the other fish. The fish in the ocean are afraid of the way he looks. Big Al tries to make friends with the others, but nothing seems to work. Finally, Big Al saves another fish from a fisherman's net. At last Big Al has friends in the ocean.

**Language Expansion:** The following questions can be used to address students' recall of this book or to expand upon concepts addressed in this book.

## Definition

1. What is a sea?
2. What is a fish?
3. What is seaweed?
4. What is a gill?
5. What is a school of fish?

## Function

1. What is the sea used for?
2. What are teeth used for?
3. What is a net used for?
4. What is a gill used for?
5. What is a friend for?

## Category

1. Name three things that live in the ocean.
2. Name three parts of a fish.
3. Name three things that Big Al tried to do to make friends.
4. Name three ways to make friends.
5. Name three of your friends.

## Description

1. Tell me three things about the ocean.
2. Tell me three things about Big Al.
3. Tell me three things about the other fish in the ocean.
4. Tell me three things about Big Al's rescue of the other fish.
5. Tell me three things about a friend.

## Vocabulary

Make a sentence using the following words.
1. sea
2. seaweed
3. gills
4. capture
5. fisherman

## Rhyming

Name a rhyming word for each word below
1. fish
2. gill
3. sea
4. net
5. Al

## Sequencing

As your students sequence the events in this story, use this list as a guide.
1. Big Al was a friendly fish, but he looked scary and he had no friends.
2. Big Al tried many things to make the other fish like him.
3. A net dropped from above, and the other fish were caught.
4. Big Al charged at the net and ripped it, and the fish escaped.
5. The fish realized how nice Big Al was and they became friends with him.

#BK-272 Year-Round Literature • ©1999 Super Duper® Publications • 1-800-277-8737 • www.superduperinc.com

# The Rainbow Fish
## by Marcus Pfister

This is a story about a rainbow fish who has beautiful, sparkling scales. The other fish in the sea are amazed at the beauty of the rainbow fish and ask him for a scale. He is unfortunately too proud and selfish, so he swims away. After time, the rainbow fish realizes he has no friends and is not happy. Then, a wise octopus tells him to give away his scales and he will be happy. He gives away his scales and finds many friends in the sea.

**Language Expansion:** The following questions can be used to address students' recall of this book or to expand upon concepts addressed in this book.

## Definition
1. What is an ocean?
2. What is a fish?
3. What is a scale?
4. What is an octopus?
5. What is a friend?

## Function
1. What is the ocean for?
2. What is a cave used for?
3. What is the octopus' ink used for?
4. What is a fin used for?
5. What is a friend for?

## Category
1. Name three things that live in the ocean.
2. Name three parts of a fish.
3. Name three things about the ocean.
4. Name three ways to make friends.
5. Name three of your friends.

## Description
1. Tell me three things about the ocean.
2. Tell me three things about the rainbow fish.
3. Tell me three things about the starfish.
4. Tell me three things about the octopus.
5. Tell me three things about a friend.

## Vocabulary
Make a sentence using the following words.
1. ocean
2. fish
3. scale
4. fin
5. friend

## Rhyming
Name a rhyming word for each word below.
1. fin
2. scale
3. cave
4. wise
5. swim

## Sequencing
As your students sequence the events in this story, use this list as a guide.
1. A rainbow fish with sparkling, silver scales lived in the ocean.
2. The other fish wanted to play with the rainbow fish, but he would just swim away.
3. The other fish asked the rainbow fish for a sparkling, silver scale, but he would not share.
4. The other fish left the rainbow fish, and he was all alone.
5. An octopus told the rainbow fish to share his scales and then he would have friends.
6. The rainbow fish shared his scales and made many friends.

# Swimmy
## by Leo Lionni

This book is about a small, black fish that lives in the ocean. A large, hungry tuna fish is roaming around, waiting to eat the small fish. So, Swimmy comes up with a plan to create one giant fish out of all of the small fish. Together, the school of fish scare the tuna fish away.

---

**Language Expansion:** The following questions can be used to address students' recall of this book or to expand upon concepts addressed in this book.

## Definition
1. What is a school of fish?
2. What is the sea?
3. What is a lobster?
4. What is seaweed?
5. What is a sea anemone?

## Function
1. What is the sea for?
2. What is swimming for?
3. What is the lobster's claw for?
4. What are fins used for?
5. What are gills used for?

## Category
1. Name three things that live in an ocean.
2. Name three sea animals that Swimmy saw in the ocean.
3. Name three parts of a fish.
4. Name three colors that a fish might be.
5. Name three things that can swim.

## Description
1. Tell me three things about the ocean.
2. Tell me three things about Swimmy.
3. Tell me three things about the tuna fish.
4. Tell me three things about the lobster.
5. Tell me three things about the eel.

## Vocabulary
Make a sentence using the following words.
1. school of fish
2. sea
3. Medusa
4. invisible
5. eel

## Rhyming
Name a rhyming word for each word below
1. eel
2. sea
3. swim
4. fins
5. fish

---

## Sequencing
As your students sequence the events in this story, use this list as a guide.
1. Swimmy is a little black fish and all his brothers and sisters are red.
2. A hungry tuna fish comes and swallows all the red fish.
3. Swimmy is lonely and swims around the ocean and meets other sea creatures.
4. Swimmy finds another school of red fish, but they are afraid of being eaten.
5. The red fish learn to swim together to look like one big fish with Swimmy as the eye, and they chase the big fish away.

#BK-272  Year-Round Literature • ©1999 Super Duper® Publications • 1-800-277-8737 • www.superduperinc.com

# Ocean Articulation and Language Games

(The following games can be used with the articulation and vocabulary word list or the literature language questions.)

## Scuba Diving Game

Make one copy of the scuba diving clothing (page 200) for each student. Color, cut out, and laminate each scuba diving outfit item. Put all of the cards in a sand bucket. After a student makes a sentence with an ocean word containing his/her sound or answers an ocean language question, the student may draw a card from the bucket. The object of the game is for each student to get the entire scuba diving outfit by the end of the session.

### Language Extension

After completing the scuba diving outfit, have each student describe each part and tell what each part is used for. Talk about why people go scuba diving.

### Team Approach

In order to win the game, each team member must complete an entire scuba diving outfit by the end of class.

## Gone Fishing Game

Photocopy, color, and laminate the "gone fishing" pattern (page 201). Turn the cards facedown. After a student makes a sentence with an ocean word containing his/her sound or answers an ocean language question, the student chooses one fish. If the fish has directions, the student must follow the directions. If the fish is blank, the student may keep the fish. The student with the most fish at the end of the game is the winner.

### Team Approach

In order to win the game, the team must earn a designated number of fish. For example, the team must have 15 fish by the end of class to win.

## Puzzle Game

Photocopy, color, laminate, and cut apart a puzzle (page 202) for every student. Put each puzzle into a separate envelope. When playing, give each student a puzzle with all of the pieces facedown. After a student makes a sentence with an ocean word containing his/her sound or answers an ocean language question, the student may turn over one piece of his/her puzzle. The object is for each student to have his/her puzzle completely together by the end of class.

### Language Extension

After completing each puzzle, allow each student to describe the ocean picture. Talk about what each is used for and how each is powered. Then, discuss the category of transportation and how some things travel in water, on land, and in the air.

## Sailboat Game

Photocopy the sailboat pattern (page 203) on yellow or blue construction paper. Cut out and laminate the sailboats. After a student makes a sentence with an ocean word containing his/her sound or answers an ocean language question, the student may draw a sailboat. The number on the back is the number of points the student receives on the score sheet for the turn. The student with the most points wins.

### Team Approach

In order to win the game, the team must earn a designated number of points. For example, the team must have 30 points by the end of class to win.

## Beach Trip Game

Make a copy of the beach trip page objects (page 204) for each student. Color the pieces, cut them apart, laminate them, and place them in a bag. Put a towel on the floor for the students to sit on during the game and tell them that you are going on a pretend beach trip. Each student must get a bucket, a shovel, sunglasses, sunscreen, a bathing suit, and flip-flops by the end of class. After a student makes a sentence with an ocean word containing his/her sound or answers an ocean language question, the student may reach into the bag and pull out one piece. If the child does not have the piece drawn, he/she may keep it for his/her trip to the beach. If the child does have the piece drawn, he/she must put it back and wait for the next turn. Whoever has all of the beach supplies first is the winner.

### Team Approach

In order to win the game, each team member must have all of the beach supplies by the end of class.

# Scuba Diving Game

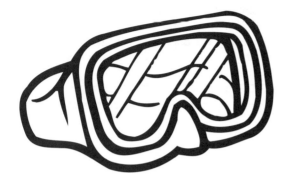
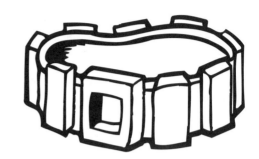
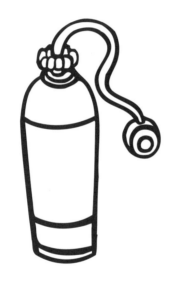
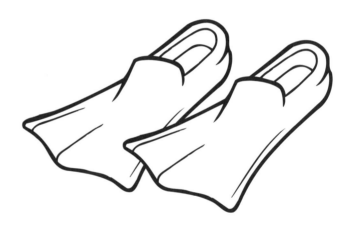
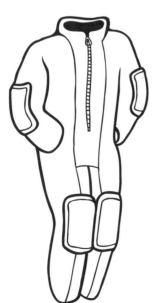
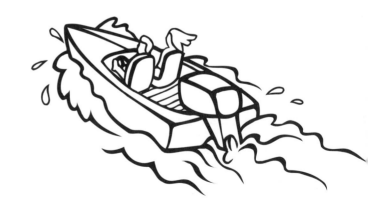

 #BK-272  Year-Round Literature  •  ©1999 Super Duper® Publications  •  1-800-277-8737  •  www.superduperinc.com

# Gone Fishing Game

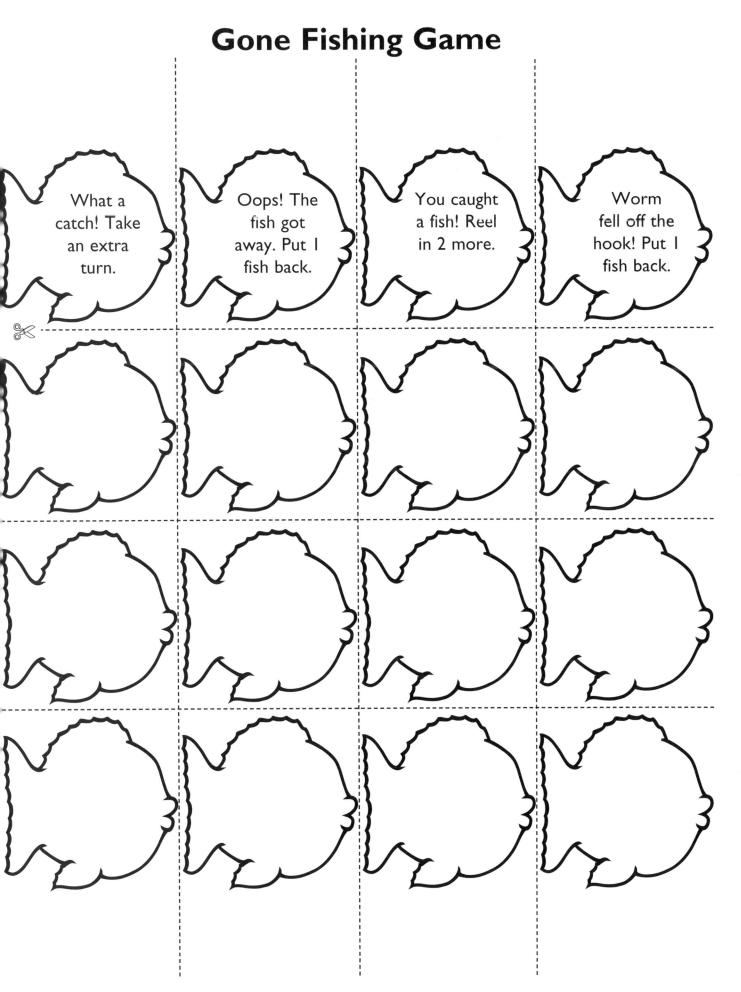

What a catch! Take an extra turn.

Oops! The fish got away. Put 1 fish back.

You caught a fish! Reel in 2 more.

Worm fell off the hook! Put 1 fish back.

# Puzzle Game

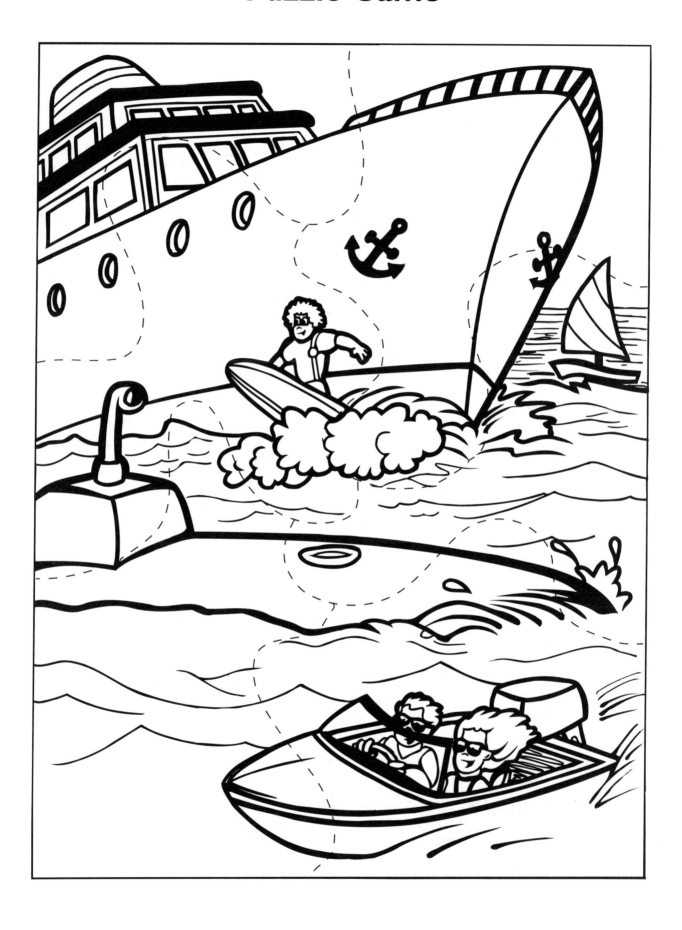

#BK-272 Year-Round Literature • ©1999 Super Duper® Publications • 1-800-277-8737 • www.superduperinc.com

# Sailboat Game

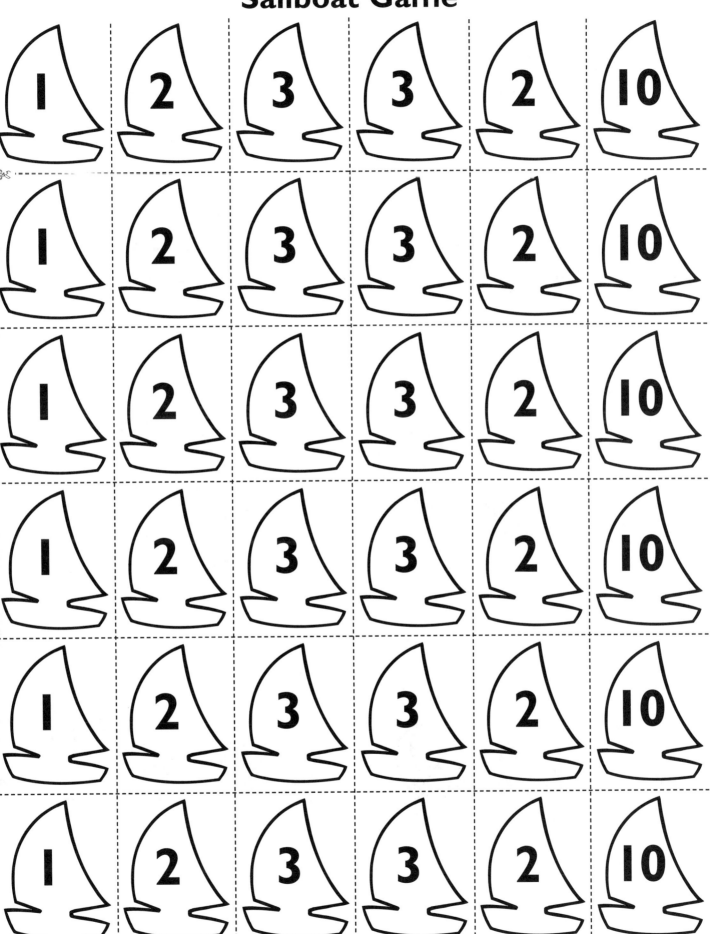

# Beach Trip Game

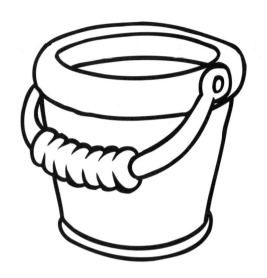

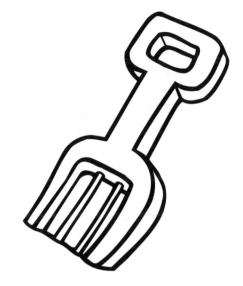

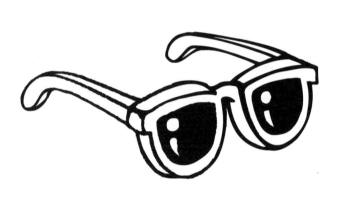

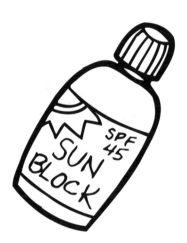

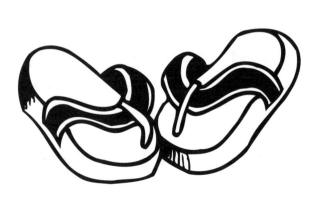

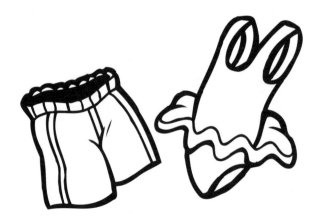

# Fishing for Good Speech

Write words with the _____ sound on each fish. Then, make a sentence with each word out loud using your good speech.

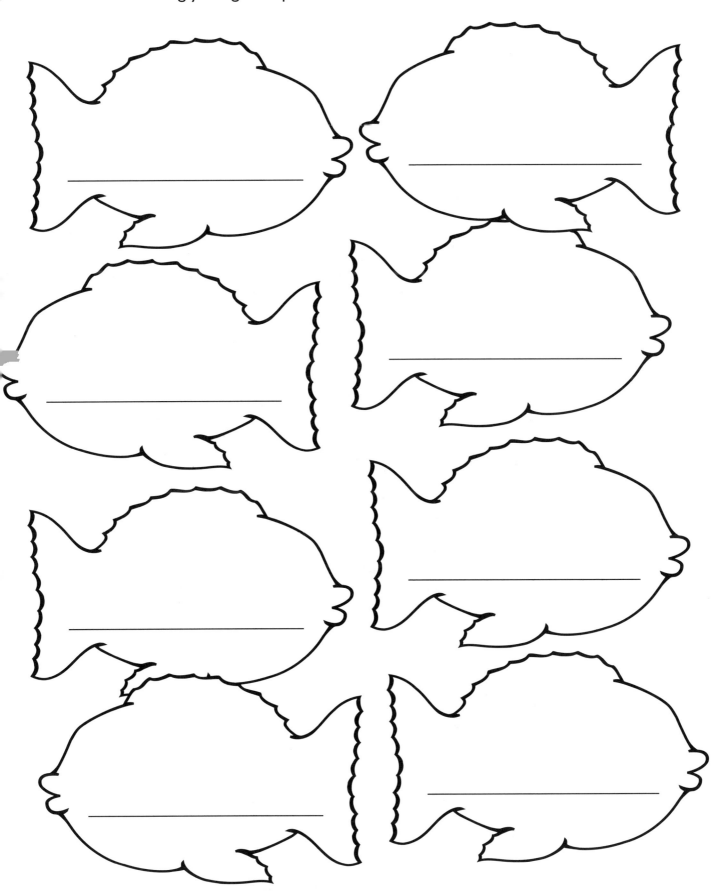

# Parts of a Fish

Can you name each part of the fish? Label the fish below with the correct word or cut out the words below and place them in the correct place.

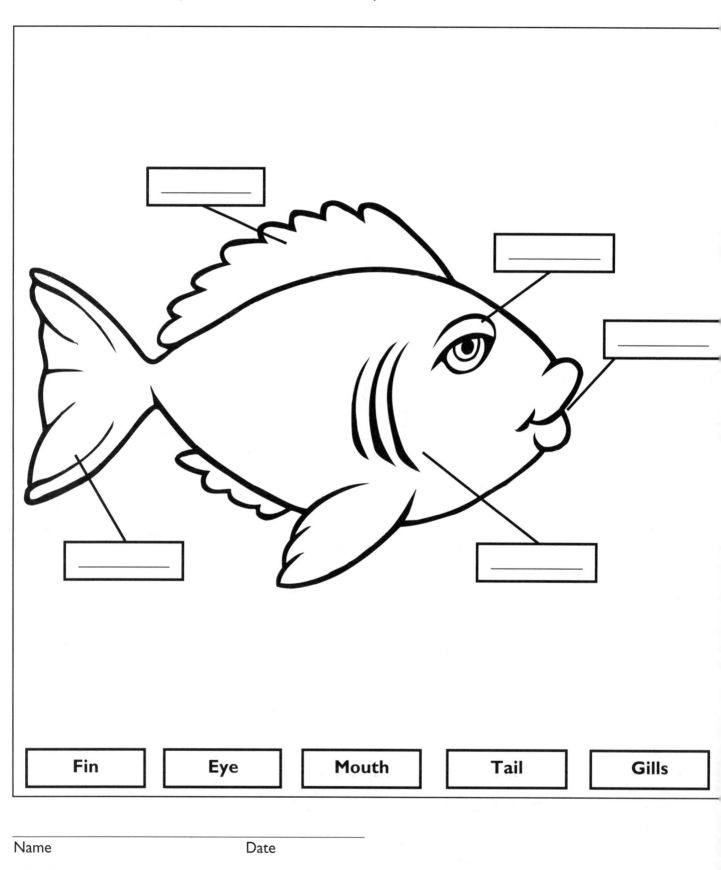

| Fin | Eye | Mouth | Tail | Gills |

Name _____ Date _____

_____

# Ocean Matching

Read each description. Then, see if you can find the picture that matches each description. Draw a line from the description to the matching picture.

| | |
|---|---|
| 1. This is a mammal, not a fish. It has a smooth body and a beaked snout. It is rather playful, intelligent, and friendly. It leaps from the water several times a minute to breathe. | |
| 2. This is a boneless sea animal. It has eight arms and a body shaped like a sack. When it becomes excited, it changes color. If it is attacked, it squirts black ink at its enemies. | |
| 3. This person searches for things in the ocean. They really like to look at the different fish and sea animals. They need special equipment. | |
| 4. This is something very heavy. It is attached to a ship or boat. When it is put into the water, it helps to keep the boat in one place. | |
| 5. This is a small fish. Its head looks similar to the head of a horse. It is covered with bony plates. It swims upright and floats on ocean currents. | |
| 6. This is a sea animal with a flat, round body surrounded by arms. Most have five arms and look like stars. If an arm breaks off, it just grows another arm. | |

Answers: 1. Dolphin, 2. Octopus, 3. Scuba Diver, 4. Anchor, 5. Seahorse, 6. Starfish

Name _____ Date _____

Speech-Language Pathologist

Helper's Signature

#BK-272  Year-Round Literature  •  ©1999 Super Duper® Publications  •  1-800-277-8737  •  www.superduperinc.com

# Granny's Candies® Board Game

## The Delicious Game of Word Meanings

Grades K-6

by Sarah Michaels and Amy Parks

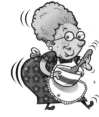

Combine the excitement of picking colorful "candy" tokens from Granny's candy jars with hundreds of opportunities to expand vocabulary building skills.

Players choose question cards and answer the questions, roll the die, and pick "candy" from the jars. The player with the most candy at the end of the game wins. You receive 672 word-meaning cards (84 for each area):

- What belongs in this group?
- What do these have in common?
- Which one doesn't belong?
- What is this used for?
- Give a describing word.
- How are they different?
- How are they alike?
- Give an action word.

Your extra ingredients include an 18″ x 18″ game board, 144 "candy" tokens, a Lesson/Activity book, a card holder, and a die.

| What belongs in this group? |
| --- |
| transportation |
| ©2002 Super Duper® Publications 10 |

| How are they alike? |
| --- |
| turtle – snail |
| ©2002 Super Duper® Publications 8 |

## Ask for Item.....................#GB-154
Granny's Candies®

## Granny's Candies® Add-On Set 2

### Vocabulary and Figurative Language

Cards & Activity Book

Grades 2-8

Use **Card and Activity Book Set 2 Vocabulary and Figurative Language** with the original **Granny's Candies®** board game. Includes 672 word-meaning cards (84 for each skill area):

- Synonyms
- Homonyms
- Heteronyms
- Similes
- Opposites
- Homophones
- Idioms
- Metaphors

Also has Lesson/Activity Book, card holder, and eight plastic baggies for storing cards.

*Note: Set 2 does not include game board, "candy tokens," and the die.

## Ask for Item..........................#GB-155
Granny's Candies® Vocabulary and Figurative Language Set 2

## Granny's Candies® Verbs Add-On Set 3

Cards & Activity Book

Grades 2-6

**Granny's Candies® Verbs Cards and Activity Book Set 3** has 672 word-meaning cards:

- Regular Past Tense
- Irregular Past Tense
- Is-Are
- Was-Were
- Has-Have
- Do-Does
- Verb+ing
- Main Verbs and Helping Verbs
- Subject-Verb Agreement
- Active-Passive Voice
- Past, Present, and Future Tense
- Contractions

Verbs Card Set 3 includes Lesson/Activity Book, card holder, and plastic baggies for storing cards.

*Note: Set 3 does not include game board, "candy tokens," and the die.

## Ask for Item........................#GB-156
Granny's Candies® Verbs Set 3

. . . . . . . . . . . . . . . . . . . . . . . . . . . . . . . . . . . . . . . . . . . . . . .

# See it, Say it® Sound Production

## Flip Book and Activities for Apraxia and More!

Book/CD-ROM Combo

Grades PreK and Up

by Jennifer Perkins Faulk and Lisa Priddy

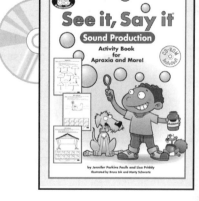

The **See it, Say it® Flip Book** contains four identical sections of illustrated cards. The cards provide a visual model of how to produce vowel and consonants at the sound, syllable, and word levels. Each card section is arranged by place of production, beginning at the front of the mouth and working towards the back. It contains worksheets and therapy activities for the illustrated cards in the See it, Say it® Flip Book. They allow the child to practice at the beginner (sound), intermediate (syllable), and advanced (word) levels. Therapy activities and reproducible mouth pictures are included to encourage carryover practice. A CD-ROM with the same worksheets and activities is also included.

## Ask for Item........#BK-317
See it, Say it® Sound Production

**Call 1-800-277-8737**
**FAX 1-800-978-7379**

**Free Shipping!**
USA and Canada

**www.superduperinc.com**
Order Anytime!

208

©2007 Super Duper® Inc.